The ECG made easy

For Churchill Livingstone

Publisher: Laurence Hunter
Project Manager: Ninette Premdas
Copy Editor: Alison Gale
Project Controller: Kay Hunston
Design: Erik Bigland

The ECG made easy

John R. Hampton DM MA DPhil FRCP FFPM FESC

Professor of Cardiology
University of Nottingham
Nottingham
UK

FIFTH EDITION

CHURCHILL
LIVINGSTONE

EDINBURGH LONDON NEW YORK PHILADELPHIA SYDNEY
TORONTO 1998

First edition 1973
Second edition 1980
Third edition 1986
Fourth edition 1992
Fifth edition 1997
   Reprinted 1998 (twice)
   Reprinted 1999
   Reprinted 2000

Standard edition ISBN 0 443 05681 1
International edition ISBN 0 443 05695 1
   Reprinted 1997
   Reprinted 1998 (twice)
   Reprinted 1999

British Library of Cataloguing in Publication Data
A catalogue record for this book is available from the British Library.

Library of Congress Cataloging in Publication Data
A catalog record available from the Library of Congress.

Medical knowledge is constantly changing. As new information becomes
available, changes in treatment, procedures, equipment and the use of
drugs become necessary. The author and the publishers have, as far as it
is possible, taken care to ensure that the information given in this text is
accurate and up to date. However, readers are strongly advised to confirm
that the information, especially with regard to drug usage, complies with
current legislation and standards of practice.

The
publisher's
policy is to use
paper manufactur
from sustainable fo

Printed in China

Preface

The ECG made easy was first published in 1973, and over a quarter of a million copies of the English language version of the first four editions have been sold. The book has been translated into German, French, Spanish, Italian, Portuguese, Polish, Indonesian and Japanese. The aims of this new edition are the same as before: the book is not intended to be a comprehensive textbook on electrophysiology, nor even of ECG interpretation, but it is designed as an introduction to the ECG for medical students, nurses and paramedics. In addition, it may provide useful revision for those who have forgotten what they learned as students.

There really is no need for the ECG to be daunting: just as most people drive a car without knowing much about engines, and gardeners do not need to be botanists, most people can make full and proper use of the ECG without getting submerged in its complexities. This book encourages the reader to accept that the ECG really is easy to understand, and that its use is just a natural extension of the history and the physical examination.

This edition of *The ECG made easy* is slightly longer than its predecessors. Some of the explanations have been lengthened, and since the aim of ECG interpretation is to help with patient management, some 'What to do' sections have been introduced. These are by no means comprehensive, but they do serve to emphasize that ECG interpretation is not an end in itself.

In a small-format text the reproduction of ECGs is inevitably difficult, and for clarity a single complex is shown for most of the 12-lead illustrations, as in the previous editions. As a step towards clinical practice, some full records have been included in this edition — although these are inevitably reduced in size compared with real records.

The ECG made easy should help the student to prepare for examinations, but for the development of clinical competence — and confidence — there is no substitute for reporting on large numbers of clinical records. Two companion texts may help those who have mastered *The ECG made easy* and want to progress further. *The ECG in practice* deals with the relationship between the patient's history and physical signs and the ECG, and with the many variations in the ECG seen in health and disease. *100 ECG problems* describes 100 clinical cases and gives their full ECGs, in a format that encourages the reader to interpret the record and decide on a course of treatment before looking at the answers.

The title *The ECG made easy* was suggested 25 years ago by the late Tony Mitchell, Foundation Professor of Medicine at the University of Nottingham. I am grateful to him and to the many people who have helped to refine the book over the years, and particularly to many students for their constructive criticisms and helpful comments, which have reinforced my belief that the ECG really is easy to understand.

John Hampton
Nottingham 1997

Contents

1. What the ECG is about   1

2. Conduction and its problems   27

3. The rhythm of the heart   53

4. Abnormalities of P waves, QRS complexes
   and T waves   92

5. Reminders   116

Index   127

CHAPTER 1

What the ECG is about

ECG stands for electrocardiogram, or electrocardiograph. In some countries, the abbreviation used is 'EKG'. Remember —

- By the time you have finished this book, you should be able to say 'The ECG is easy to understand'.
- Most abnormalities of the ECG are amenable to reason.

WHAT TO EXPECT FROM THE ECG

Clinical diagnosis depends mainly on a patient's history, and to a lesser extent on the physical examination. The ECG can provide evidence to support a diagnosis, and in some cases it is crucial for patient management. It is, however, important to see the ECG as a tool, and not as an end in itself.

The ECG is essential for the diagnosis, and therefore management, of abnormal cardiac rhythms. It helps with the diagnosis of the cause of chest pain, and the proper use of thrombolysis in treating myocardial infarction depends upon it. It can help with the diagnosis of the cause of breathlessness.

With practice, interpreting the ECG is a matter of pattern recognition. However, the ECG can be analysed from first principles if a few simple rules and basic facts are remembered. This chapter is about these rules and facts.

THE ELECTRICITY OF THE HEART

The contraction of any muscle is associated with electrical changes called 'depolarization', and these changes can be detected by electrodes attached to the surface of the body. Since all muscular contraction will be detected, the electrical changes associated with contraction of the heart muscle will only be clear if the patient is fully relaxed and no skeletal muscles are contracting.

Although the heart has four chambers, from the electrical point of view it can be thought of as having only two, because the two atria contract together and then the two ventricles contract together.

The wiring diagram of the heart

The electrical discharge for each cardiac cycle normally starts in a special area of the right atrium called the 'sinoatrial (SA) node'. Depolarization then spreads through the atrial muscle fibres. There is a delay while the depolarization spreads through another special area in the atrium, the 'atrioventricular node' (also called the 'AV node', or sometimes just 'the node'). Thereafter, the electrical discharge travels very rapidly, down specialized conduction tissue: first a single pathway, the 'bundle of His', which then divides in the septum between the ventricles into right and left bundle branches. The left bundle branch itself divides into two. Within the mass of ventricular muscle, conduction spreads somewhat more slowly, through specialized tissue called 'Purkinje fibres'.

The rhythm of the heart

As we shall see later, electrical activation of the heart can sometimes begin in places other than the SA node. The word 'rhythm' is used to refer to the part of the heart which is controlling the activation sequence. The normal heart rhythm, with electrical activation beginning in the SA node, is called 'sinus rhythm'.

THE SHAPE OF THE ECG

The muscle mass of the atria is small compared with that of the ventricles, and the electrical change accompanying the contraction of the atria is therefore small. Contraction of the atria is associated with the ECG wave called 'P'. The ventricular mass is large, and so there is a large deflection of the ECG when the ventricles are depolarised. This is called the 'QRS' complex. The 'T' wave of the ECG is associated with the return of the ventricular mass to its resting electrical state ('repolarization').

The basic shape of the normal ECG is:

The letters P, Q, R, S and T were selected in the early days of ECG history, and were chosen arbitrarily. The P, Q, R, S and T deflections are all called waves; the Q, R and S waves together make up a complex; and the interval between the S wave and the T wave is called the ST 'segment'.

The different parts of the QRS complex are labelled as follows. If the first deflection is downward, it is called a Q wave.

An upward deflection is called an R wave,

— whether it is preceded by a Q wave or not.

Any deflection below the baseline following an R wave is called an S wave,

— whether there has been a preceding Q wave or not.

Times and speeds

ECG machines record changes in electrical activity by drawing a trace on a moving paper strip. All ECG machines run at a standard rate and use paper with standard-sized squares. Each large square (5 mm) represents 0.2 seconds, so there are five large squares per second, and 300 per minute. So an ECG event, such as a QRS complex, occurring once per large square is occurring at a rate of 300 per minute. The heart rate can be calculated rapidly by remembering this sequence: If the R–R interval is:

1	large square, the rate is				300 beats/min
2	″ squares,	″	″	″	150 beats/min
3	″	″	″	″	″ 100 beats/min
4	″	″	″	″	″ 75 beats/min
5	″	″	″	″	″ 60 beats/min
6	″	″	″	″	″ 50 beats/min

1 small square represents   1 large square represents
0.04 s   0.2 s

5 large squares represent 1 s
1 QRS complex per s
Heart rate = 60 per min

Just as the length of paper between R waves gives the heart rate, so the distance between the different parts of the P-QRS-T complex shows the time taken for conduction of the electrical discharge to spread through the different parts of the heart.

The PR interval is measured from the beginning of the P wave to the begining of the QRS complex, and is the time taken for excitation to spread from the SA node, through the atrial muscle and the AV node, down the bundle of His and into ventricular muscle.

The normal PR interval is 0.12–0.2 s (120–200 ms), represented by three to five small squares. Most of the time is taken up by delay in the AV node. If the PR interval is very short, either the atria have been depolarized from close to the AV node, or there is abnormally fast conduction from the atria to the ventricles.

PR 0.16 s   **QRS 0.10 s**

The duration of the QRS complex shows how long excitation takes to spread through the ventricles. The QRS duration is normally 0.12 s (represented by three small squares) or less, but any abnormality of conduction takes longer, and causes widened QRS complexes.

PR 0.16 s   **QRS 0.20 s**

RECORDING AN ECG

The word 'lead' sometimes causes confusion. Sometimes it is used to mean the pieces of wire that connect the patient to the ECG recorder. Properly, a lead is an electrical picture of the heart.

The electrical signal from the heart is detected at the surface of the body through five electrodes, which are joined to the ECG recorder by wires. One electrode is attached to each limb and one is held by suction to the front of the chest and moved to different positions. Good electrical contact between the electrodes and skin is essential. It may be necessary to shave the chest.

The ECG recorder compares the electrical activity detected in the different electrodes, and the electrical picture so obtained is called a 'lead'. The different comparisons 'look at' the heart from different directions. For example, when the recorder is set to 'lead I' it is comparing the electrical events detected by the electrodes attached to the right and left arms. Each lead gives a different view of the electrical activity of the heart, and so a different ECG pattern. Properly, each ECG pattern should be called 'lead . . .', but often the word 'lead' is omitted.

It is not necessary to remember which electrodes are involved in which leads, but it is essential that the electrodes are properly attached, with the wires labelled 'LA' and 'RA' connected to the left and right arms respectively and those labelled 'LL' and 'RL' to the left and right legs respectively. As we shall see, the ECG is made up of characteristic pictures, and the record as a whole is almost uninterpretable if the electrodes are wrongly attached.

The 12-lead ECG

ECG interpretation is easy if you remember the directions from which the various leads look at the heart. The six 'standard' leads, which are recorded from the electrodes attached to the limbs, can be thought of as looking at the heart in a vertical plane (that is, from the sides or the feet).

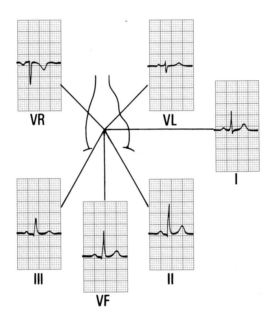

Leads I, II and VL look at the left lateral surface of the heart, III and VF at the inferior surface, and VR looks at the right atrium.

The V lead is attached to the chest wall by means of a

suction electrode, and recordings are made from six
positions, overlying the 4th and 5th rib spaces as
shown.

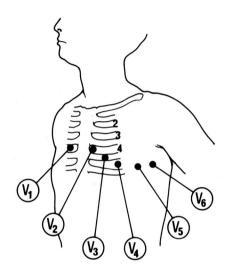

The six numbered V leads look at the heart in a
horizontal plane, from the front and the left side.

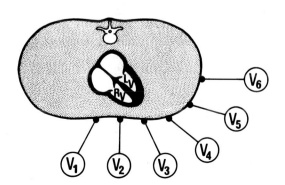

Thus leads V_1 and V_2 look at the right ventricle, V_3 and V_4 look at the septum between the ventricles and the anterior wall of the left ventricle, and V_5 and V_6 look at the anterior and lateral walls of the left ventricle. As with the limb leads, the chest leads each show a different ECG pattern. In each lead the pattern is characteristic, being similar in different individuals who have normal hearts.

Calibration

A limited amount of information is provided by the height of the P waves, QRS complexes and T waves, provided the machine is properly calibrated. For example, small complexes may indicate a pericardial effusion, and tall R waves may indicate left ventricular hypertrophy (see Chapter 4). A standard signal of 1 mV should move the stylus vertically 1 cm (two large squares), and this 'calibration' signal should be included with every record.

CALIBRATION

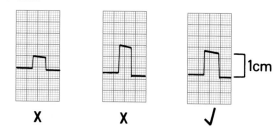

X   X   ✓

Making a recording

When making a recording:

1. The patient must lie down and relax (to prevent muscle tremor)
2. Connect up the limb electrodes, making certain that they are applied to the correct limb
3. Calibrate the record with the 1 mV signal
4. Record the six standard leads — three or four complexes are sufficient for each
5. Record the six V leads.

THE SHAPE OF THE QRS COMPLEX

We now need to consider why the ECG has a characteristic appearance in each lead.

The QRS complex in the limb leads

The ECG machine is arranged so that when a depolarization wave spreads towards a lead the stylus moves upwards, and when it spreads away from the lead the stylus moves downwards.

Depolarization spreads through the heart in many directions at once, but the shape of the QRS complex shows the average direction in which the wave of depolarization is spreading through the ventricles.

If the QRS complex is predominantly upward, or positive (that is, the R wave is greater than the S wave), the depolarization is moving towards that lead.

If predominantly downward, or negative (S wave greater than R wave), the depolarization is moving away from that lead.

When the depolarization wave is moving at right angles to the lead, the R and S waves are of equal size.

Q waves have a special significance, which we shall discuss later.

The cardiac axis

VR and II look at the heart from opposite directions. Seen from the front, the depolarization wave normally spreads through the ventricles from 11 o'clock to 5 o'clock, so the deflections in VR are normally mainly downward (negative) and in II mainly upward (positive).

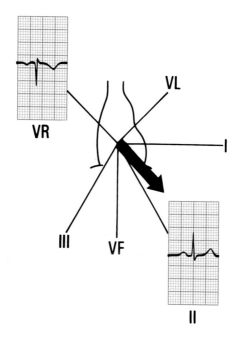

The average direction of spread of the depolarization wave through the ventricles as seen from the front is called the 'cardiac axis'. It is useful to decide whether this axis is in a normal direction or not. The direction of the axis can be derived most easily from the QRS complex in leads I, II and III.

A normal 11 o'clock–5 o'clock axis means that the depolarizing wave is spreading towards leads I, II and III and is therefore associated with a predominantly upward deflection in all these leads; the deflection will be greater in II than in I or III.

NORMAL AXIS

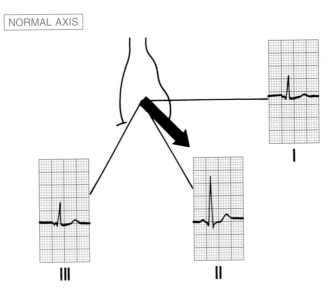

If the right ventricle becomes hypertrophied, the axis will swing towards the right: the deflection in I becomes negative (predominantly downward) and the deflection in III will become more positive (predominantly upward). This is called 'right axis deviation'. It is associated mainly with pulmonary conditions that put a strain on the right side of the heart, and with congenital heart disorders.

RIGHT AXIS DEVIATION

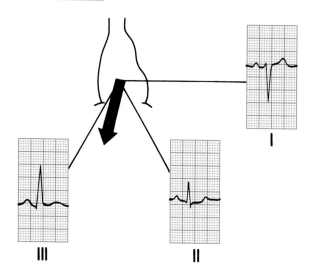

When the left ventricle becomes hypertrophied, the axis may swing to the left, so that the QRS complex becomes predominantly negative in III. 'Left axis deviation' is not significant until the QRS deflection is also predominantly negative in II, and the problem is usually due to a conduction defect rather than to increased bulk of the left ventricular muscle (see Ch. 2).

LEFT AXIS DEVIATION

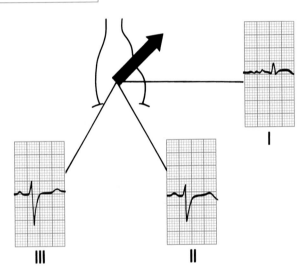

Right and left axis deviation in themselves are seldom significant — minor degrees occur in long, thin individuals and in short, fat individuals respectively. However, the presence of axis deviation should alert you to look for other signs of right and left ventricular hypertrophy (see Ch. 4).

An alternative explanation of the cardiac axis

Some people find the cardiac axis a difficult concept, and an alternative approach to working it out may be helpful.

The cardiac axis is at right angles (90°) to the lead in which the R and S waves are of equal size.

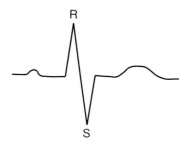

It is, of course, likely that the axis will not be precisely at right angles to any of the leads, but will be somewhere between two of them. The axis points towards any lead where the R wave is larger than the S wave. It points away from any lead where the S wave is larger than the R wave.

The cardiac axis is sometimes measured in degrees, though this is not clinically particularly useful. Lead I is taken as looking at the heart from 0°; lead II from +60°; VF from +90°; and III from +120°. VL and VR are said to look from −30° and −150° respectively.

The normal cardiac axis is in the range −30° to +90°. For example, if in lead II the size of the R wave equals that of the S wave, the axis is at right angles to lead II. In theory, the axis could be at either −30° or +150°. However, in these circumstances lead I will usually show an R wave greater than the S wave, so the axis must point towards lead I rather than lead III. Therefore the true axis is at −30° — this is the limit of normality towards what is called the 'left'. If in lead II the S wave is greater than the R wave, the axis is at

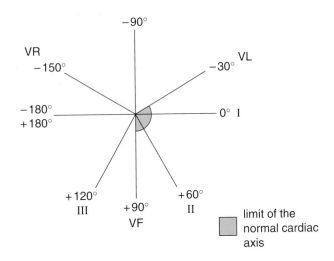

limit of the normal cardiac axis

an angle of greater than −30°, and left axis deviation is present. Similarly, if the size of the R wave equals that of the S wave in lead I, the axis is at right angles to lead I or at +90°. This is the limit of normality towards the 'right'. If the S wave is greater than the R wave in lead I, the axis is at an angle of greater than +90°, and right axis deviation is present.

The QRS complex in the V leads

The shape of the QRS complex in the chest (V) leads is determined by two things:

- The septum between the ventricles is depolarized before the walls of the ventricles, and the depolarization wave spreads across the septum from left to right.
- In the normal heart there is more muscle in the wall of the left ventricle than in that of the right ventricle, and so the left ventricle exerts more influence on the ECG pattern than does the right ventricle.

   Leads V_1 and V_2 look at the right ventricle; leads V_3 and
V_4 look at the septum; and leads V_5 and V_6 at the left
ventricle (see diagram on p. 9).
   In a right ventricular lead the deflection is first upwards
(R wave) as the septum is depolarized. In a left ventricular
lead the opposite pattern is seen: there is a small
downward deflection ('septal' Q wave).

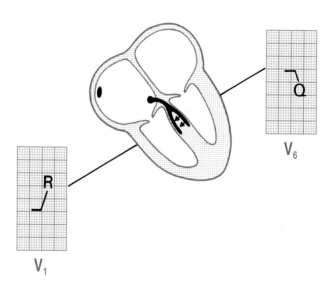

In a right ventricular lead (V_1 and V_2) there is then a downward deflection (S wave) as the main muscle mass is depolarized — the electrical effects in the bigger left ventricle (in which depolarization is spreading away from a right ventricular lead) outweighing those in the smaller right ventricle (in which depolarization is moving towards a right ventricular lead). In a left ventricular lead there is an upward deflection (R wave) as the ventricular muscle is depolarized.

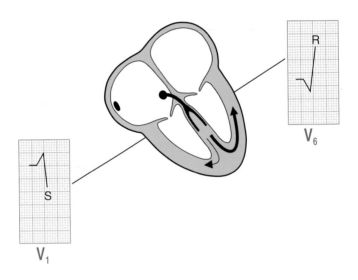

When the whole of the myocardium is depolarized the ECG returns to baseline.

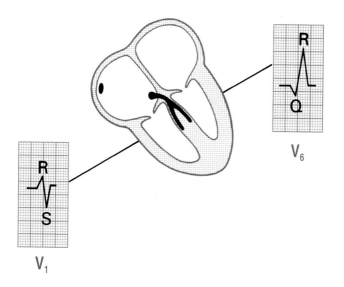

The QRS complex in the chest leads shows a progression from V_1, where it is predominantly downward, to V_6, where it is predominantly upward. The 'transition point', where the R and S waves are equal, indicates the position of the interventricular septum.

If the right ventricle is enlarged, and occupies more of the precordium than is normal, the transition point will move from its normal position of V_3/V_4 to V_4/V_5 or sometimes V_5/V_6. Seen from below, the heart can be thought of as having rotated in a clockwise direction. 'Clockwise rotation' in the ECG is characteristic of chronic lung disease.

HOW TO REPORT AN ECG

You now know enough about the ECG to understand the basis of a report. This should take the form of a description, followed by an interpretation.

The description should always be given in the same sequence:

1. Rhythm
2. Conduction intervals
3. Cardiac axis
4. A description of the QRS complexes
5. A description of the ST segments and T waves.

Reporting a series of totally normal findings is possibly pedantic, and in real life is frequently not done. However, you must think about all the findings every time you interpret an ECG.

ECG INTERPRETATION

The interpretation indicates whether the record is normal or abnormal: if abnormal, the underlying pathology needs to be identified.

We shall come to abnormal ECGs in later chapters, but first try to report the two following 12-lead records.

This ECG shows:

- Sinus rhythm, rate 110 per minute
- PR interval normal, at 140 ms
- QRS duration normal, at 120 ms
- Normal cardiac axis
- Normal QRS complexes
- Normal T waves (an inverted T wave in lead VR is normal).

Interpretation: Normal ECG.

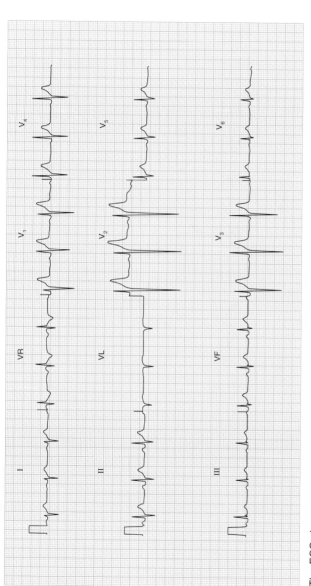

The ECG shows:
- Sinus rhythm rate 75 per minute
- PR interval 200 ms
- QRS duration 120 ms
- Right axis deviation (prominent S wave in lead I)
- Normal QRS complexes
- Normal ST segments and T waves.

Interpretation:
Normal ECG, apart from right axis deviation, which could be normal in a tall thin person. Unfortunately, there are a lot of minor variations in the ECG which are consistent with perfectly normal hearts. Recognizing the limits of normality is one of the main difficulties of ECG interpretation.

THINGS TO REMEMBER

1. The ECG results from electrical changes associated with activation first of the atria and then of the ventricles.
2. Atrial activation causes the P wave.
3. Ventricular activation causes the QRS complex. If the first deflection is downward it is a Q wave. Any upward deflection is an R wave. A downward deflection after an R wave is an S wave.

4. When the depolarization wave spreads towards a lead, the deflection is predominantly upward. When the wave spreads away from a lead, the deflection is predominantly downward.
5. The six limb leads (I, II, III, VR, VL and VF) look at the heart from the sides and the feet in a vertical plane.
6. The cardiac axis is the average direction of spread of depolarization as seen from the front, and is estimated from leads I, II and III.
7. The chest or V leads look at the heart from the front and the left side in a horizontal plane. V_1 is positioned over the right ventricle, V_6 over the left ventricle.
8. The septum is depolarized from the left side to the right.
9. The left ventricle exerts more influence on the ECG than the right ventricle, in a normal heart.

CHAPTER 2
Conduction and its problems

We have already seen that electrical activation normally begins in the sinoatrial node, and that a wave of depolarization spreads outwards through the atrial muscle to the atrioventricular node, and thence down the His bundle and its branches to the ventricles. The conduction of this wave front can be delayed or blocked at any point. However —

- Conduction problems are simple to analyse provided you keep the wiring diagram of the heart constantly in mind.

SA node —

AV node —

Bundle of His

Lt. bundle branch

Rt. bundle branch

We can think of conduction problems in the order in which the depolarization wave normally spreads from the sinoatrial node — AV node, His bundle, and bundle branches. Remember in all that follows that we are assuming depolarization begins in the normal way in the SA node.

The rhythm of the heart is best interpreted from whichever ECG lead shows it most clearly. This is usually, but not always, lead II or lead V$_1$. You can assume that all the 'rhythm strips' in this book were recorded from one of these leads.

CONDUCTION PROBLEMS IN THE AV NODE AND HIS BUNDLE

The time taken for the spread of depolarization from the SA node to the ventricular muscle is shown by the PR interval (see Ch. 1), and is not normally greater than 0.2 s (one large square). Interference with the conduction process causes the ECG phenomenon called 'heart block'.

First degree heart block

If each wave of depolarization that originates in the SA node is conducted to the ventricles, but there is delay somewhere along the conduction pathway, then the PR interval is prolonged. This is called 'first degree heart block'.

FIRST DEGREE BLOCK

PR 0.36 s

Note: One P wave per QRS complex
PR interval 0.36 s.

First degree heart block is not in itself important, but it may be a sign of coronary artery disease, acute rheumatic carditis, digitalis toxicity or electrolyte disturbances.

Second degree heart block

Sometimes excitation completely fails to pass through the AV node or the bundle of His. When this occurs intermittently, 'second degree heart block' is said to exist. There are three variations of this:

1. Most beats are conducted with a constant PR interval, but occasionally there is an atrial contraction without a subsequent ventricular contraction. This is called the 'Mobitz Type 2' phenomenon.

SECOND DEGREE BLOCK (Mobitz type 2)

Note: PR interval of the conducted beats is constant
One P wave is not followed by a QRS complex, and
here second degree block is occurring.

2. There may be progressive lengthening of the PR interval and then failure of conduction of an atrial beat, followed by a conducted beat with a shorter PR interval and then a repetition of this cycle. This is the 'Wenckebach' phenomenon.

SECOND DEGREE BLOCK (Wenckebach type)

Note: Progressive lengthening of PR interval
One non-conducted beat
Next conducted beat has a shorter PR interval than the preceding conducted beat.

3. There may be alternate conducted and non-conducted atrial beats (or one conducted atrial beat and then two non-conducted beats), giving twice (or three times) as many P waves as QRS complexes. This is called '2:1' ('2 to 1') (or '3:1' ('3 to 1')) conduction.

SECOND DEGREE BLOCK (2:1 type)

Note: Two P waves per QRS complex
Normal, and constant, PR interval in the conducted beats.

It is important to remember that, as with any other rhythm, a P wave may only show itself as a distortion of a T wave.

SECOND DEGREE BLOCK (2:1 type)

Note: P wave in the T wave can be identified because of its regularity.

The underlying causes of second degree heart block are the same as those of first degree block. The Wenckebach phenomenon is usually benign, but Mobitz Type 2 block and 2:1 block may herald 'complete,' or 'third degree', heart block.

Third degree heart block

Complete heart block (third degree block) is said to occur when atrial contraction is normal but no beats are conducted to the ventricles. When this occurs the ventricles are excited by a slow 'escape mechanism' (see Ch. 3), from a depolarizing focus within the ventricular muscle.

THIRD DEGREE (COMPLETE) BLOCK

Note: P wave rate 90 per minute

QRS complex rate 36 per minute

No relationship between P waves and QRS complexes

Abnormally-shaped QRS complexes because of abnormal spread of depolarization from a ventricular focus.

Complete heart block may occur as an acute phenomenon in patients with myocardial infarction (when it is usually transient) or it may be a chronic state, usually due to fibrosis around the bundle of His. It may also be caused by the block of both bundle branches.

CONDUCTION PROBLEMS IN THE RIGHT AND LEFT BUNDLE BRANCHES — BUNDLE BRANCH BLOCK

If the depolarization wave reaches the interventricular septum normally, then the interval between the beginning of the P wave and the first deflection in the QRS complex (the PR interval) will be normal. However, if there is abnormal conduction through either the right or left bundle branches ('bundle branch block') there will be a delay in the depolarization of part of the ventricular muscle. The extra time taken for depolarization of the whole of the ventricular muscle causes widening of the QRS complex.

In the normal heart, the time taken for the depolarization wave to spread from the interventricular septum to the furthest part of the ventricles is not more than 0.12 s, represented by three small squares of ECG paper. If the QRS duration is greater than 0.12 s, then conduction within the ventricles must have occurred by an abnormal and therefore slow pathway.

Although a wide QRS complex can indicate bundle branch block, widening also occurs if depolarization begins within the ventricular muscle itself (see Ch. 3). Remember that in sinus rhythm with bundle branch block, normal P waves are present with a constant PR interval. We shall see that this is not the case with rhythms beginning in the ventricles.

Block of both bundle branches has the same effect as block of the His bundle, and causes complete (third degree) heart block.

Right bundle branch block (RBBB) often indicates problems in the right side of the heart, but RBBB patterns with a QRS complex of normal duration are quite common in healthy people.

Left bundle branch block (LBBB) is always an indication of heart disease, usually of the left side. It is important to recognize that bundle branch block is present, because LBBB prevents any further interpretation of the cardiogram, and RBBB can make interpretation difficult.

The mechanism underlying the ECG patterns of right and left bundle branch block can be worked out from first principles. Remember (see Ch. 1):

- The septum is normally depolarized from left to right.
- The left ventricle, having the greater muscle mass, exerts more influence on the ECG than does the right ventricle.
- Excitation spreading towards a lead causes an upward deflection within the ECG.

Right bundle branch block

No conduction occurs down the right bundle branch, but the septum is depolarized from the left side as usual, causing an R wave in a right ventricular lead (V₁) and a small Q wave in a left ventricular lead (V₆).

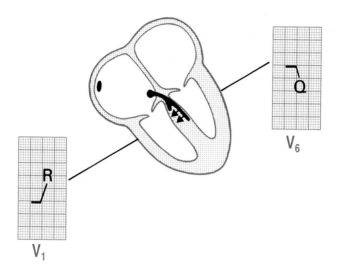

Excitation then spreads to the left ventricle, causing an S wave in V_1 and an R wave in V_6.

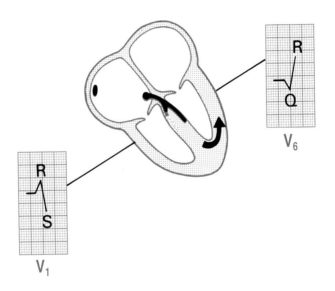

It takes longer than in a normal heart for excitation to reach the right ventricle because of the failure of the normal conducting pathway. The right ventricle therefore depolarizes after the left. This causes a second R wave (R^1) in V_1, and a wide and deep S wave in V_6.

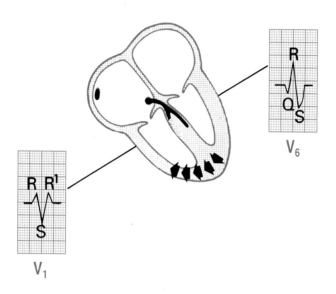

An 'RSR^1' pattern, but with a QRS complex of normal width (less than 120 ms) is sometimes called 'partial right bundle branch block'. It is seldom of significance, and can be considered to be a normal variant.

Left bundle branch block

If conduction down the left bundle branch fails, the septum becomes depolarized from right to left, causing a small Q wave in V_1, and an R wave in V_6.

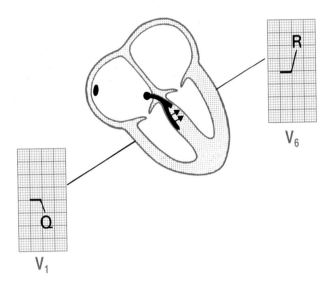

The right ventricle is depolarized before the left, so despite the smaller muscle mass there is an R wave in V₁ and an S wave (often appearing only as a notch) in V₆.

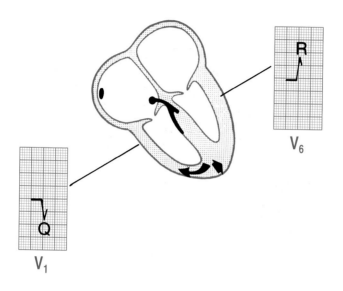

Subsequent depolarization of the left ventricle causes an S wave in V_1 and another R wave in V_6.

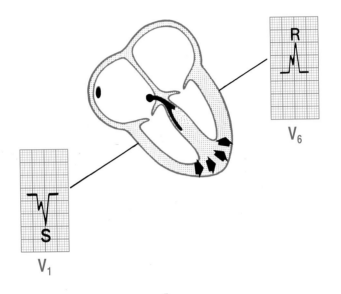

What to remember

RBBB is best seen in lead V_1 where there is an RSR[1] pattern.

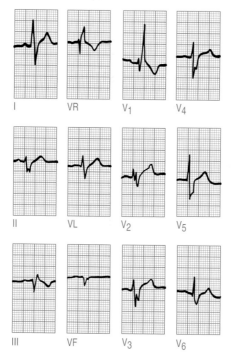

Note: Sinus rhythm
PR interval normal
Wide QRS complexes
RSR[1] pattern in lead V_1
Deep, slurred S wave in lead V_6.

LBBB is best seen in lead V_6, where there is a broad complex with a notched top, resembling the letter 'M' and known as an 'M' pattern. The complete picture, with a 'W' pattern in lead V_1, is often not fully developed.

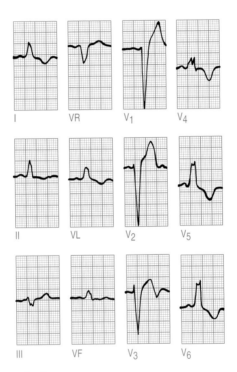

I VR V_1 V_4

II VL V_2 V_5

III VF V_3 V_6

Note: Sinus rhythm
PR interval normal
Wide QRS complexes
M pattern in QRS complexes, best seen in leads V_4–V_6
Inverted T waves in leads I, VL, V_4–V_6 (T wave inversion in the anterior lateral leads is characteristic of LBBB, see p. 109).

CONDUCTION PROBLEMS IN THE DISTAL PARTS OF THE LEFT BUNDLE BRANCH

At this point it is worth considering in a little more detail the anatomy of the branches of the His bundle. The right bundle branch has no main divisions but the left bundle branch has two — the anterior and posterior 'fascicles'. The depolarization wave therefore spreads into the ventricles by three routes, shown below:

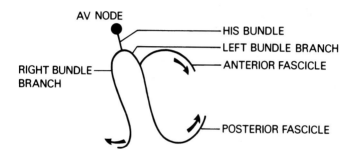

The cardiac axis (see Ch. 1) depends on the average direction of depolarization of the ventricles. Since the left ventricle contains more muscle than the right, it has more influence on the cardiac axis.

If the anterior fascicle of the left bundle branch fails to conduct, the left ventricle has to be depolarized through the posterior fascicle and so the cardiac axis rotates upwards.

LEFT AXIS
DEVIATION

Left axis deviation is therefore due to left anterior fascicular block, or 'left anterior hemiblock'.

The posterior fascicle of the left bundle is not often selectively blocked, but if this does occur the ECG shows right axis deviation.

When the right bundle branch is blocked, the cardiac axis usually remains normal, because there is normal depolarization of the left ventricle with its large muscle mass.

RBBB

However, if both the right bundle branch and the left anterior fascicle are blocked, the ECG shows right bundle branch block and left axis deviation (LAD).

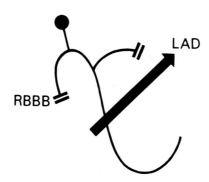

This is sometimes called 'bifascicular block', and this particular ECG pattern obviously indicates widespread damage to the conducting system.

If the right bundle branch and both fascicles of the left bundle branch are blocked, complete heart block occurs just as if the main His bundle had failed to conduct.

WHAT TO DO

Always remember that it is the patient who should be treated, not the ECG. Relief of symptoms always comes first. However, some general points can be made about the action that might be taken if the ECG shows conduction abnormalities.

First degree block

- Often seen in normal people
- Think about acute myocardial infarction and acute rheumatic fever as possible causes
- No specific action needed.

Second degree block

- Usually indicates heart disease; often seen in acute myocardial infarction
- Mobitz Type 2 and Wenckebach block do not need specific treatment
- 2:1 block may indicate a need for temporary or permanent pacing, especially if the ventricular rate is slow.

Third degree block

- Always indicates conducting tissue disease — more often fibrosis than ischaemic
- A pacemaker is needed — temporary in the context of acute infarction, otherwise permanent.

Right bundle branch block

- Think about an atrial septal defect
- No specific treatment.

Left bundle branch block

- Think about aortic stenosis and ischaemic disease
- If the patient is asymptomatic, no action is needed
- If the patient has recently had severe chest pain, LBBB may indicate an acute myocardial infarction and thrombolysis should be considered.

Left axis deviation

- Think about left ventricular hypertrophy
- No action needed.

Left axis deviation and right bundle branch block

- Indicates severe conducting tissue disease
- No specific treatment needed
- Pacemaker required if the patient has symptoms suggestive of intermittent complete heart block.

ECG INTERPRETATION

Now report the four following 12-lead ECG records which illustrate conduction problems.

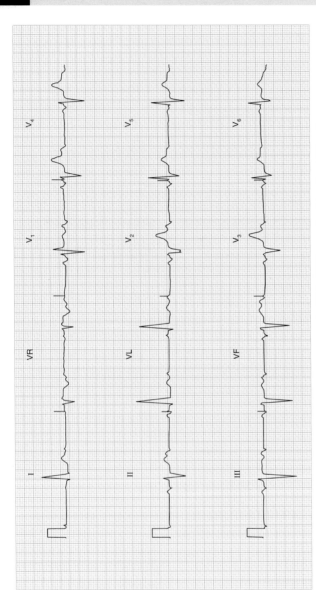

The ECG shows:
- Sinus rhythm
- Alternate conducted and non-conducted beats
- Normal PR interval in the conducted beats
- Left axis deviation (deep S waves in both leads II and III)
- Wide QRS complex (duration 160 ms)
- RSR[1] pattern in lead V[1].

Interpretation:
Second degree (2:1) block with left anterior hemiblock and right bundle branch block, indicating severe conducting tissue disease.

The ECG shows:
- Sinus rhythm, but no P waves are conducted
- Right axis deviation
- Broad QRS complexes (duration 160 ms)
- Right bundle branch block pattern.

Interpretation:
Complete heart block with a ventricular escape pattern. The cause cannot be determined, though in most patients it results from fibrosis of the bundle of His.

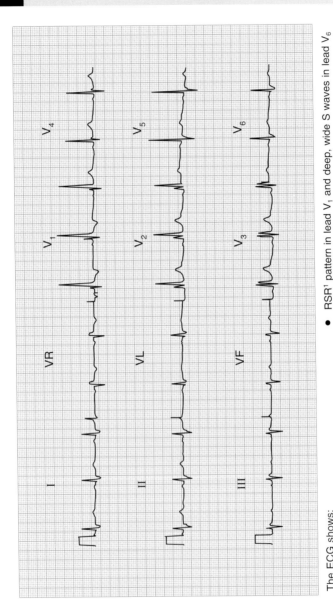

The ECG shows:

- Sinus rhythm rate 75 per minute
- Normal PR interval
- Normal cardiac axis
- Wide QRS complexes (160 ms)
- RSR¹ pattern in lead V_1 and deep, wide S waves in lead V_6
- Normal ST segments and T waves.

Interpretation:
Sinus rhythm with right bundle branch block.

The ECG shows:

- Sinus rhythm rate 100 per minute
- Normal PR interval
- Normal cardiac axis
- Wide QRS complexes (160 ms)

- M pattern in the QRS complexes, best seen in leads I, VL, V₅, V₆
- Inverted T waves in leads I, II, VL.

Interpretation:
Sinus rhythm with left bundle branch block.

THINGS TO REMEMBER

1. Depolarization normally begins in the SA node, and spreads to the ventricles via the AV node, the His bundle, the right and left branches of the His bundle, and the anterior and posterior fascicles of the left bundle branch.

2. A conduction abnormality can develop at any of these points.

3. Conduction problems in the AV node and His bundle may be partial (first and second degree block) or complete (third degree block).

4. If conduction is normal through the AV node, the His bundle and one of its branches, but is abnormal in the other branch, bundle branch block exists and the QRS complex is wide.

5. The ECG pattern of RBBB and LBBB can be worked out if you remember (a) that the septum is depolarized first from left to right; (b) that V_1 looks at the right ventricle and V_6 at the left ventricle; and (c) that when depolarization spreads towards an electrode the stylus moves upwards.

6. If you can't remember all this, remember that RBBB has an RSR[1] pattern in V_1, while LBBB has an M pattern in V_6.

7. Block of the anterior division or fascicle of the left bundle branch causes left axis deviation.

CHAPTER 3
The rhythm of the heart

So far we have only considered the spread of depolarization
that follows the normal activation of the sinoatrial (SA) node.
When depolarization begins in the SA node the heart is
said to be in sinus rhythm. Depolarization can, however,
begin in other places. Then the rhythm is named after the
part of the heart where the depolarization sequence
originates, and an 'arrhythmia' is said to be present.
Remember —

- Abnormalities of cardiac rhythm are easy to work out.
  The two things to look at are the P waves and the
  width of the QRS complexes.

When attempting to analyse a cardiac rhythm remember:

- Atrial contraction is associated with the P wave of the
  ECG
- Ventricular contraction is associated with the QRS
  complex
- Atrial contraction normally precedes ventricular
  contraction, and there is normally one atrial contraction
  per ventricular contraction (i.e. there should be as
  many P waves as there are QRS complexes).

THE INTRINSIC RHYTHMICITY OF THE HEART

Most parts of the heart can depolarize spontaneously and

rhythmically, and the rate of contraction of the ventricles will be controlled by the part of the heart that is depolarizing most frequently. The SA node normally has the highest frequency of discharge. Therefore the rate of contraction of the ventricles will equal the rate of discharge of the SA node.

The rate of discharge of the SA node is influenced by the vagus nerves, and reflexes originating in the lung also affect the heart rate. Changes in heart rate associated with respiration are normally seen in young people, and this is called 'sinus arrhythmia'.

In the diagram below, and in the other diagrams in this chapter, the star indicates the part of the heart where the activation sequence began.

SINUS ARRHYTHMIA

Note: One P wave per QRS complex
Constant PR interval
Progressive beat-to-beat change in R–R interval.

A slow sinus rhythm ('sinus bradycardia') is associated with trained athletes, fainting attacks, hypothermia, and myxoedema, and it is often seen immediately after a heart attack. A fast sinus rhythm ('sinus tachycardia') is associated with exercise, fear, pain, haemorrhage and thyrotoxicosis. There is no particular rate that is called 'bradycardia' or 'tachycardia' — these are merely descriptive terms.

Abnormal cardiac rhythms can begin in three places — the atrial muscle; the region around the AV node (this rhythm is called 'nodal' or more properly, 'junctional'); or the ventricular muscle. In the diagram below the stars suggest specific points within the atrial and ventricular muscles at which electrical activation might begin, but abnormal rhythms can begin anywhere within the atrial or ventricular muscle.

SA node
Atrial muscle
AV node
Ventricular muscle

Sinus rhythm, atrial rhythm, and junctional rhythm together constitute the 'supraventricular' rhythms.

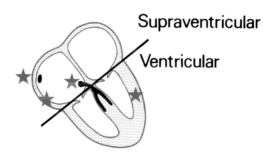

Supraventricular

Ventricular

In the supraventricular rhythms, the depolarization wave spreads to the ventricles in the normal way via the His bundle and its branches. The QRS complex is therefore normal, and is the same whether depolarization was initiated by the SA node, the atrial muscle, or the junctional region.

In ventricular rhythms, on the other hand, the depolarization wave spreads through the ventricles by an abnormal, and therefore slower, pathway through the Purkinje fibres. The QRS complex is therefore wide and abnormal. Repolarization is also abnormal, so the T wave is of abnormal shape.

Remember:

1. Supraventricular rhythms have narrow QRS complexes
2. Ventricular rhythms have wide QRS complexes
3. The only exception to this rule occurs when there is a supraventricular rhythm with right or left bundle branch block.

TYPES OF ABNORMAL RHYTHM

Abnormal rhythms arising in the atrial muscle, the junctional region or the ventricular muscle can be slow and sustained (bradycardias); or they can occur as early single beats ('extrasystoles'); or they can be fast and sustained (tachycardias). When activation of the atria or ventricles is totally disorganized, 'fibrillation' is said to occur. We shall consider each of these types of rhythm in turn.

The escape rhythms — the bradycardias

It is clearly advantageous if different parts of the heart are able to initiate the depolarization sequence, because this gives the heart a series of 'fail-safe' mechanisms that will keep it going if the SA node fails to depolarize, or if conduction of the depolarization wave is blocked. However, the protective mechanisms must normally be inactive if competition between normal and abnormal sites of spontaneous depolarization is to be avoided. This is achieved by the secondary sites having a lower intrinsic frequency of depolarization than the SA node.

The heart is controlled by whichever site is spontaneously depolarizing most frequently: normally this is the SA node, and it gives a normal heart rate of about 70 per minute. If the SA node fails to depolarize, control will be assumed by a focus either in the atrial muscle or in the region around the AV node (the junctional region), both of which have spontaneous depolarization frequencies of about 50 per minute. If these fail, or if conduction through the His bundle is blocked, a ventricular focus will take over and give a ventricular rate of about 30 per minute.

These slow and protective rhythms are called escape rhythms, because they occur when secondary sites for initiating depolarization escape from their normal inhibition by the more active SA node.

Escape rhythms are not primary disorders, but are the response to problems higher in the conducting pathway. They are commonly seen in the acute phase of a heart attack, when they may be associated with sinus bradycardia. It is important not to try to suppress an escape rhythm, because without it the heart might stop altogether.

Atrial escape

If the rate of depolarization of the SA node slows down and
a focus in the atrium takes over control of the heart, the
rhythm is described as 'atrial escape'. Atrial escape beats
can occur singly.

ATRIAL ESCAPE

Note: After one sinus beat the SA node fails to depolarize.
After a delay an abnormal P wave is seen because
excitation of the atrium has begun somewhere away
from the SA node. The abnormal P wave is followed
by a normal QRS complex, because excitation has
spread normally down the His bundle. The remaining
beats show a return to sinus arrhythmia.

Nodal or junctional escape

If the region around the AV node takes over as the focus of depolarization, the rhythm is called 'nodal', or more properly, 'junctional' escape.

NODAL (JUNCTIONAL) ESCAPE

Note: Sinus rate 100 per minute; junctional escape rhythm (following arrow) at 70 per minute
No P waves in junctional beats (indicates either no atrial contraction or P wave lost in QRS complex)
Normal QRS complexes.

Ventricular escape

'Ventricular escape' most commonly occurs when conduction between the atria and ventricles is interrupted. Ventricular escape rhythm is classically associated with complete heart block.

COMPLETE HEART BLOCK

P   QRS

Note: Regular P waves (normal atrial depolarization)
P wave rate 145 per minute
QRS complexes highly abnormal because of abnormal conduction through ventricular muscle
QRS (ventricular escape) rate 15 per minute
No relationship between P waves and QRS complexes.

Ventricular escape rhythms can occur without complete heart block. Ventricular escape beats can be single.

VENTRICULAR ESCAPE

Note: After three sinus beats, the SA node fails to discharge. No atrial or nodal escape occurs. After a pause there is a single wide and abnormal QRS complex (arrow) with an abnormal T wave. A ventricular focus controls the heart for one beat and sinus rhythm is then restored.

The rhythm of the heart can occasionally be controlled by a ventricular focus with an intrinsic frequency of discharge faster than that seen in complete heart block. The rhythm is called 'accelerated idioventricular rhythm'. This is often associated with acute myocardial infarction.

ACCELERATED IDIOVENTRICULAR RHYTHM

Note: After three sinus beats, the SA node fails to depolarize. An escape focus in the ventricle takes over, causing a regular rhythm of 75 per minute with wide QRS complexes and abnormal T waves.

Although the appearance of the ECG is similar to that of ventricular tachycardia (see p. 75), accelerated idioventricular rhythm is benign and should not be treated. Ventricular tachycardia should not be diagnosed unless the heart rate exceeds 120 per minute.

EXTRASYSTOLES

Any part of the heart can depolarize earlier than it should, and the accompanying heart beat is called an extrasystole. The term 'ectopic' is sometimes used to indicate that depolarization originated in an abnormal location, and the term 'premature contraction' means the same thing.

The ECG appearance of an extrasystole arising in either the atrial muscle, the junctional or nodal region, or the ventricular muscle, is the same as that of the corresponding escape beat — the difference is that an extrasystole comes early and an escape beat comes late.

Atrial extrasystoles have abnormal P waves. In a junctional extrasystole either there is no P wave at all, or it appears immediately before or immediately after the QRS complex. The QRS complexes of atrial and junctional extrasystoles are, of course, the same as those of sinus rhythm.

ATRIAL AND JUNCTIONAL (NODAL)
EXTRASYSTOLES

Sinus | Atrial
  Junctional

Note: This record shows sinus rhythm with junctional and atrial extrasystoles
A junctional extrasystole has no P wave
An atrial extrasystole has an abnormally-shaped P wave.
Sinus, junctional and atrial beats have identical QRS complexes — conduction in and beyond the bundle of His is normal

Ventricular extrasystoles, however, have abnormal QRS complexes, which are typically wide but can be of almost any shape. Ventricular extrasystoles are common and are usually of no importance. However, when they occur early in the T wave of a preceding beat they can induce ventricular fibrillation (see p. 80), and are thus potentially dangerous.

VENTRICULAR EXTRASYSTOLE

with R on T phenomenon

Note: Upper trace shows five sinus beats, then an early beat with a wide QRS complex and an abnormal T wave: this is a ventricular extrasystole. In the lower trace, the ventricular extrasystoles occur (arrows) at the peak of the T waves of the preceding sinus beats: this is the 'R on T' phenomenon.

It may, however, not be as easy as this, particularly if a beat of supraventricular origin is conducted abnormally to the ventricles (bundle branch block, see Ch. 2). It is advisable to get into the habit of asking five questions every time an ECG is being analysed:

1. Does an early QRS complex follow an early P wave? If so, it must be an atrial extrasystole.
2. Can a P wave be seen anywhere? A junctional extrasystole may cause the appearance of a P wave very close to, and even after, the QRS complex because excitation is conducted both to the atria and to the ventricles.
3. Is the QRS complex the same shape throughout (i.e. has it the same initial direction of deflection as the normal beat, and has it the same duration)? Supraventricular beats look the same, ventricular beats look different.
4. Is the T wave the same way up as in the normal beat? In supraventricular beats, it is the same way up; in ventricular beats, it is inverted.
5. Does the next P wave after the extrasystole appear at an expected time? In both supraventricular and ventricular extrasystoles there is a ('compensatory') pause before the next heart beat, but a supraventricular extrasystole usually upsets the normal periodicity of the SA node, so that the next SA node discharge (and P wave) comes late.

The effects of supraventricular and ventricular extrasystoles on the following P wave are seen in the next two examples.

A supraventricular extrasystole resets the P wave cycle.

SUPRAVENTRICULAR EXTRASYSTOLE

No P wave

Expected P wave

P

Note: Three sinus beats are followed by a junctional extrasystole. No P wave is seen at the expected time and the next P wave is late.

A ventricular extrasystole, on the other hand, does not affect the SA node, so the next P wave appears at the predicted time.

VENTRICULAR EXTRASYSTOLE

Note: Three sinus beats are followed by a ventricular extrasystole. No P wave is seen after this beat, but the next P wave arrives on time.

THE TACHYCARDIAS — THE FAST RHYTHMS

Foci in the atria, the junctional (AV nodal) region, and ventricles may fire repeatedly, causing a sustained tachycardia. The criteria already described can be used to decide the origin of the arrhythmia, and as before the most important thing is to try to identify a P wave.

Supraventricular tachycardias

Atrial tachycardia (abnormal focus in the atrium)

In atrial tachycardia, the atria contract faster than 150 per minute.

ATRIAL TACHYCARDIA

Note: After three sinus beats, atrial tachycardia develops at a rate of 150 per minute. P waves can be seen superimposed on the T waves of the preceding beats. The QRS complexes have the same shape as those of the sinus beats.

The AV node cannot conduct atrial rates of discharge greater than about 200 per minute. If the atrial rate is faster than this, 'atrioventricular block' occurs, with some P waves not followed by QRS complexes. The difference between this sort of atrioventricular block and second degree heart block is that in atrioventricular block associated with a tachycardia the AV node is functioning properly — it is preventing the ventricles from being activated at a fast (and therefore inefficient) rate. In first, second or third degree block associated with sinus rhythm the AV node and/or the His bundle are not conducting normally.

Atrial flutter

When the atrial rate is greater than 250 per minute, and there is no flat baseline between the P waves, 'atrial flutter' is present.

ATRIAL FLUTTER (4:1)

P

Note: P waves can be seen at a rate of 300 per minute, giving a sawtoothed appearance. There are four P waves per QRS complex, and ventricular activation is perfectly regular at 75 per minute.

When atrial tachycardia or atrial flutter is associated with 2:1 block, you need to look carefully to recognize the extra P waves.

ATRIAL FLUTTER (2:1)

P

Note: Atrial flutter with an atrial rate of 300 per minute is present, and there is 2:1 block, giving a ventricular rate of 150 per minute. The first of the two P waves associated with each QRS complex can be mistaken for the T wave of the preceding beat, but P waves can be identified by their regularity. In this trace, T waves cannot be clearly identified.

Carotid sinus pressure may have a useful therapeutic effect on supraventricular tachycardias, and is always worth trying because it may make the nature of the arrhythmia more obvious. Carotid sinus pressure activates a reflex that leads to vagal stimulation of the SA and AV nodes. This causes a reduction of the frequency of discharge of the SA node, and an increase in the delay of conduction in the AV node. It is the latter which is important in the diagnosis and treatment of arrhythmias. Carotid sinus pressure slows the ventricular rate in some supraventricular arrhythmias and completely abolishes others, but it has no effect on ventricular arrhythmias.

ATRIAL FLUTTER WITH CAROTID SINUS
PRESSURE (CSP)

Note: In this case, carotid sinus pressure (applied during the period indicated by the arrows) has increased the block between atria and ventricles and has made it obvious that the underlying rhythm is atrial flutter.

Junctional (nodal) tachycardia

If the area around the AV node depolarizes frequently, the P waves may be seen very close to the QRS complexes (as with the corresponding extrasystoles), or may not be seen at all. The QRS complex is of normal shape because, as with the other supraventricular arrhythmias, the ventricles are activated via the bundle of His in the normal way.

JUNCTIONAL (NODAL) TACHYCARDIA

SINUS RHYTHM

Note: In the upper trace there are no P waves, and the QRS complexes are completely regular. The lower trace is from the same patient, in sinus rhythm. The QRS complexes have essentially the same shape as those of the junctional tachycardia.

Ventricular tachycardias

If a focus in the ventricular muscle depolarizes with high frequency (causing, in effect, rapidly repeated ventricular extrasystoles), the rhythm is called 'ventricular tachycardia'. Excitation has to spread by an abnormal path through the ventricular muscle, and the QRS complex is therefore wide and abnormal.

VENTRICULAR TACHYCARDIA

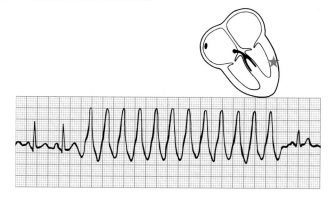

Note: After two sinus beats, the rate increases to 150 per minute. The QRS complexes become broad, and the T waves are difficult to identify. The final beat shows a return to sinus rhythm.

Remember that wide and abnormal complexes are also seen with bundle branch block.

SINUS RHYTHM WITH LEFT BUNDLE BRANCH BLOCK

Note: Sinus rhythm: each QRS complex is preceded by a P wave, with a constant PR interval. The QRS complexes are wide and the T waves are inverted. This trace was recorded from lead V_6, and the M pattern and inverted T wave characteristic of LBBB are easily identified.

How to distinguish between ventricular tachycardia and supraventricular tachycardia with bundle branch block

It is essential to remember that the patient's clinical state — whether good or bad — does not help to differentiate between the two possible causes of a tachycardia with broad QRS complexes. If a patient with an acute myocardial infarction has a broad-complex tachycardia it will almost always be a ventricular tachycardia; but a patient with episodes of such a tachycardia without an infarction could be having either a ventricular tachycardia or a supraventricular tachycardia with bundle branch block. Under such circumstances the following points may be helpful:

1. Finding P waves and seeing how they relate to the QRS complexes is always the key to identifying arrhythmias. Always look carefully at a full 12-lead ECG.
2. If possible, compare the QRS complex during the tachycardia with that during sinus rhythm. If the patient has bundle branch block when in sinus rhythm, the QRS complex during the tachycardia will have the same shape as during normal rhythm.
3. If the QRS complex is wider than four small squares (160 ms), the rhythm will probably be ventricular in origin.
4. Left axis deviation during the tachycardia usually indicates a ventricular origin, as does a change of axis compared with a record taken during sinus rhythm.
5. If during the tachycardia the QRS complex is very irregular, the rhythm is probably atrial fibrillation with bundle branch block (see below).

FIBRILLATION

All the arrhythmias discussed so far have involved the synchronous contraction of all the muscle fibres of the atria or of the ventricles, albeit at abnormal speeds. When individual muscle fibres contract independently they are said to be 'fibrillating'. Fibrillation can occur in the atrial or ventricular muscle.

When the atrial muscle fibres contract independently there are no P waves on the ECG, only an irregular line. At times there may be flutter-like waves for 2 or 3 seconds. The AV node is continuously bombarded with depolarization waves of varying strength, and depolarization spreads at irregular intervals down the bundle of His. The AV node conducts in an 'all or none' fashion, so that the depolarization waves passing into the His bundle are of constant intensity. However, these waves are irregular and the ventricles therefore contract irregularly. Because conduction into and through the ventricles is by the normal route, each QRS complex is of normal shape.

ATRIAL FIBRILLATION

Lead II

Lead V₁

Note: No P waves — irregular baseline
Irregular QRS complexes
Normally-shaped QRS complexes
In lead V₁ waves can be seen with some
resemblance to those seen in atrial flutter — this is
common in atrial fibrillation.

When the ventricular muscle fibres contract independently, no QRS complex can be identified and the ECG is totally disorganized.

VENTRICULAR FIBRILLATION

As the patient will usually have lost consciousness by the time you have realized that the change in the ECG pattern is not just due to a loose connection, the diagnosis is easy.

WOLFF-PARKINSON-WHITE (WPW) SYNDROME

The only normal electrical connection between the atria and ventricles is the His bundle. Some people, however, have an extra or 'accessory' conducting bundle. Accessory bundles form a direct connection between atrium and ventricle, usually on the left side of the heart, and in the accessory bundle there is no AV node to delay conduction. A depolarization wave therefore reaches the ventricle early and 'pre-excitation' occurs. The PR interval is short and the QRS complex shows an early slurred upstroke called a 'delta wave'. The second part of the QRS complex is normal, as conduction through the His bundle catches up with the pre-excitation.

The only clinical importance of this anatomical abnormality is that it can cause paroxysmal tachycardia. Depolarization can spread down the His bundle and back up the accessory pathway, and so reactivate the atrium. A 're-entry' circuit is thus set up, and a sustained tachycardia occurs.

WOLFF-PARKINSON-WHITE
SYNDROME

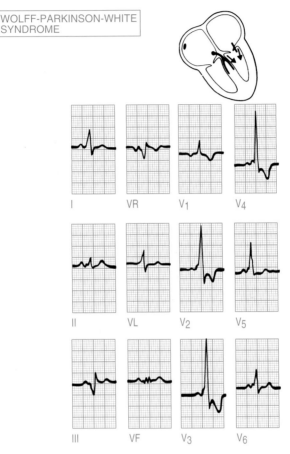

I	VR	V₁	V₄
II	VL	V₂	V₅
III	VF	V₃	V₆

Note: The 12-lead ECG shows sinus rhythm
The PR interval is short
There is a slurred upstroke of the QRS complex
The dominant R wave in V_1 and the inverted T wave
in the anterior chest leads are characteristic of the
WPW syndrome.

SUSTAINED TACHYCARDIA IN THE WPW
SYNDROME

Note: During re-entry tachycardia, no P waves can be seen.

THE ORIGINS OF TACHYCARDIAS

We have considered the tachycardias up to now as if all
were due to an increased spontaneous frequency of
depolarization of some part of the heart. While such an
'enhanced automaticity' certainly accounts for some
tachycardias, others are due to re-entry circuits within the
heart muscle. It is not possible to distinguish enhanced
automaticity from re-entry tachycardia on standard ECGs,
but fortunately this differentiation has no practical
importance.

WHAT TO DO

Accurate interpretation of the ECG is an essential part of
arrhythmia management. Although this book is not intended
to discuss therapy in any detail, it seems appropriate to
outline some simple approaches to patient management
that logically follow interpretation of an ECG recording:

1. For fast or slow sinus rhythm, treat the underlying cause,
   not the rhythm itself.

2. Extrasystoles rarely need treatment.
3. In patients with acute heart failure or low blood pressure due to a tachycardia, DC cardioversion should be considered early on.
4. Patients with any bradycardia that is affecting the circulation can be treated with atropine, but if this is ineffective they will need temporary or permanent pacing.

PACEMAKER

Note: Occasional P waves are visible, but are not related to the QRS complexes. The QRS complexes are preceded by a brief spike, representing the pacemaker stimulus. The QRS complexes are broad, because pacemakers stimulate the right ventricle and cause 'ventricular' beats.

5. The first treatment for any abnormal tachycardia is carotid sinus pressure. This should be performed with the ECG running, and may help make the diagnosis:

- Sinus tachycardia — carotid sinus pressure causes temporary slowing of the heart rate
- Atrial and junctional tachycardia — carotid sinus pressure may terminate the arrhythmia or may have no effect
- Atrial flutter — carotid sinus pressure usually causes a temporary increase in block (for example, from 2:1 to 3:1)

- Atrial fibrillation and ventricular tachycardia — carotid sinus pressure has no effect.

6. Narrow complex tachycardias should be treated initially with adenosine.
7. Wide complex tachycardias should be treated initially with lignocaine.

ECG INTERPRETATION

Now report on the following four 12-lead ECG records and consider what treatment might be indicated.

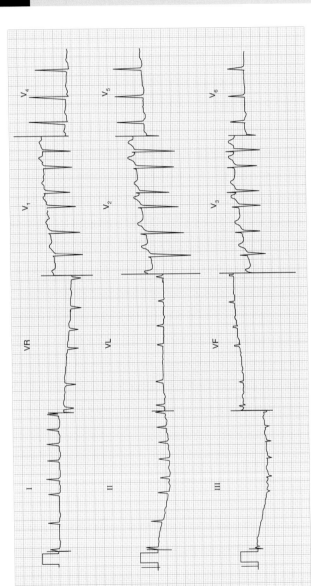

The ECG shows:
- No P waves
- Irregular baseline
- Irregular QRS complexes, rate varying between 80 and 180 per minute
- Narrow QRS complexes of normal shape

- Depressed ST segments in leads V_5–V_6
- Normal T waves.

Interpretation:
Atrial fibrillation. The ST segment depression suggests digitalis effect (see p. 109).

Treatment: Digoxin is correct treatment

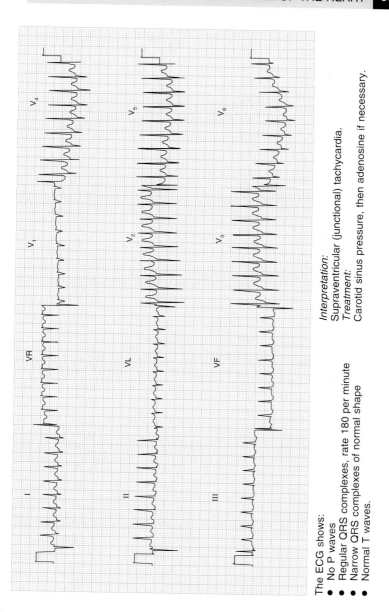

The ECG shows:

- No P waves
- Regular QRS complexes, rate 180 per minute
- Narrow QRS complexes of normal shape
- Normal T waves.

Interpretation:
Supraventricular (junctional) tachycardia.
Treatment:
Carotid sinus pressure, then adenosine if necessary.

The ECG shows:
- P waves at 300 per minute (most easily seen in leads II and VR)
- Regular QRS complexes, rate 150 per minute
- Narrow QRS complexes of normal shape
- Normal T waves (best seen in the V leads; in the limb leads it is difficult to distinguish between T and P waves).

Interpretation: Atrial flutter with 2:1 block.
Treatment, try in order:
   Carotid sinus pressure
   Adenosine
   Flecainide
   May need DC cardioversion.

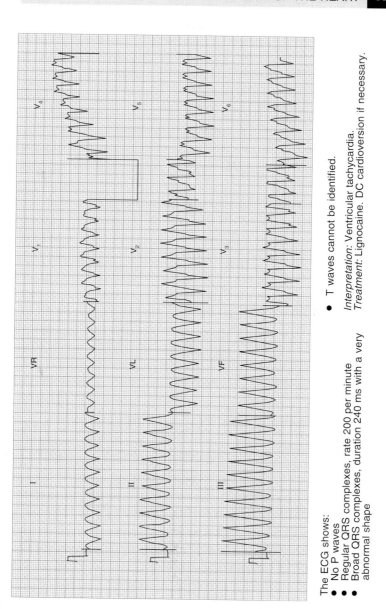

The ECG shows:
- No P waves
- Regular QRS complexes, rate 200 per minute
- Broad QRS complexes, duration 240 ms with a very abnormal shape
- T waves cannot be identified.

Interpretation: Ventricular tachycardia.
Treatment: Lignocaine. DC cardioversion if necessary.

THINGS TO REMEMBER

1. Most parts of the heart are capable of spontaneous depolarization.
2. Abnormal rhythms can arise in the atrial muscle, the region around the AV node (the junctional region) and in the ventricular muscle.
3. Escape rhythms are slow and are protective.
4. Occasional early depolarization of any part of the heart causes an extrasystole.
5. Frequent depolarization of any part of the heart causes a tachycardia.
6. Asynchronous contraction of muscle fibres in the atria or ventricles is called fibrillation.
7. Apart from the rate, the ECG pattern of an escape rhythm, an extrasystole and a tachycardia arising in any one part of the heart are the same.
8. All supraventricular rhythms have normal QRS complexes provided there is no bundle branch block (see Ch. 2).
9. Ventricular rhythms cause wide and abnormal QRS complexes, and abnormal T waves.

Recognizing ECG abnormalities is to a large extent like recognizing an elephant — once seen, never forgotten. However, in cases of difficulty it is helpful to ask the following questions, referring to Table 3.1:

1. Is the abnormality occasional or sustained?
2. Are there any P waves?
3. Are there as many QRS complexes as P waves?
4. Are the ventricles contracting regularly or irregularly?
5. Is the QRS complex of normal shape?
6. What is the ventricular rate?

Table 3.1 gives a flow diagram for analysing rhythm and conduction abnormalities.

Table 3.1 Recognizing ECG abnormalities

Abnormality	P wave	P:QRS ratio	QRS regularity	QRS shape	QRS rate	Rhythm
Occasional (i.e. extrasystoles)	Present	P:QRS = 1:1	Regular	Normal	Normal	Supraventricular
Sustained				Abnormal		Ventricular
			Regular	Normal	Normal	Sinus rhythm
					160/min +	Atrial tachycardia
			Slightly irregular	Normal	Normal	Sinus arrhythmia
			Regular	Normal	Slow	Atrial escape
		More Ps than QRSs	Regular	Normal	Fast	Atrial tachycardia with block
					Slow	2° heart block
	Absent		Regular	Abnormal	Slow	Complete heart block
				Normal	Fast	Nodal tachycardia
					Slow	Nodal escape
				Abnormal	Fast	Nodal tachycardia with bundle branch block
			Slightly irregular	Abnormal	Fast	Ventricular tachycardia
			Very irregular	Normal		Atrial fibrillation
		QRS absent			Any speed	Ventricular fibrillation or standstill

CHAPTER 4
Abnormalities of P waves, QRS complexes and T waves

When interpreting an ECG, identify the rhythm first. Then ask the following questions — always in the same sequence:

1. Are there any abnormalities of the P wave?
2. What is the cardiac axis? (Look at the QRS complex in leads, I, II, III — and at Chapter 1 if necessary)
3. Is the QRS complex of normal duration?
4. Are there any other abnormalities in the QRS complex — particularly, are there any abnormal Q waves?
5. Is the ST segment raised or depressed?
6. Is the T wave normal?

Remember —

1. The P wave can only be normal, unusually tall, or unusually broad
2. The QRS complex can only have three abnormalities — it can be too broad, too tall, and it may contain an abnormal Q wave
3. The ST segment can only be normal, elevated or depressed
4. The T wave can only be the right way up or the wrong way up.

ABNORMALITIES OF THE P WAVE

Apart from alterations of the shape of the P wave associated with rhythm changes, there are only two important abnormalities:

1. Anything that causes the right atrium to become hypertrophied (such as tricuspid valve stenosis or pulmonary hypertension) causes the P wave to become peaked.

RIGHT ATRIAL HYPERTROPHY

2. Left atrial hypertrophy (usually due to mitral stenosis) causes a broad and bifid P wave.

LEFT ATRIAL HYPERTROPHY

ABNORMALITIES OF THE QRS COMPLEX

The normal QRS complex has four characteristics:

1. Its duration is no greater than 0.12 s (three small squares)
2. In a right ventricular lead (V_1), the S wave is greater than the R wave
3. In a left ventricular lead (V_5 or V_6), the height of the R wave is less than 25 mm
4. Left ventricular leads may show Q waves due to septal depolarization, but these are less than 1 mm across and less than 2 mm deep.

Abnormalities of the width of the QRS complex

QRS complexes are abnormally wide in the presence of bundle branch block (see Ch. 2) or when depolarization is initiated by a focus in the ventricular muscle (see Ch. 3). In either case, the increased width indicates that depolarization has spread through the ventricles by an abnormal and therefore slow pathway.

Increased height of the QRS complex

An increase of muscle mass in either ventricle will lead to increased electrical activity, and to an increase in the height of the QRS complex.

Right ventricular hypertrophy

Right ventricular hypertrophy is best seen in the right ventricular leads (especially V₁). Since the left ventricle does not have its usual dominant effect on the QRS shape, the complex becomes upright (i.e. the height of the R wave exceeds the depth of the S wave) — this is nearly always abnormal. There will be a deep S wave in V₆.

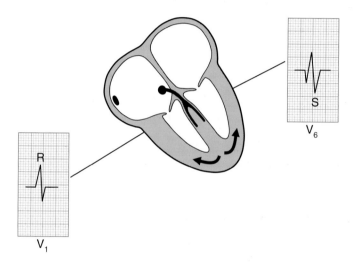

Right ventricular hypertrophy is usually accompanied by right axis deviation (see Ch. 1), by a peaked P wave (right atrial hypertrophy), and in severe cases by inversion of the T waves in V_1 and V_2, and sometimes V_3 or even V_4.

RIGHT VENTRICULAR HYPERTROPHY

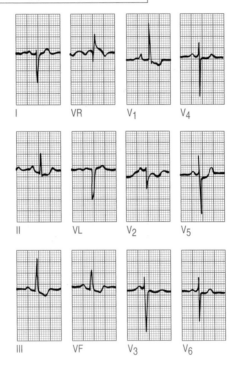

Note: Sinus rhythm
Peaked P wave in V_1
Right axis deviation (deep S wave in lead I)
Tall R wave in V_1
Deep S wave in V_6
Clockwise rotation (no septal complex seen)
Inverted T waves in V_1 and V_2.

Pulmonary embolism

In pulmonary embolism the ECG may show features of right ventricular hypertrophy, although in many cases there is nothing abnormal other than a sinus tachycardia. When a pulmonary embolus is suspected, look for:

1. Peaked P waves
2. Right axis deviation (S waves in I)
3. Tall R waves in V_1
4. Right bundle branch block
5. Inverted T waves in V_1 (normal), spreading across to V_2 or V_3
6. A shift of transition point to the left, so that the R wave equals the S wave in V_5 or V_6 rather than in V_3 or V_4. A deep S wave will persist in V_6
7. Curiously, a 'Q' wave in lead III resembling an inferior infarction (see p. 102).

However, do not hesitate to treat the patient if the clinical picture suggests pulmonary embolism but the ECG does not show the classical pattern of right ventricular hypertrophy. If in doubt, treat the patient with an anticoagulant.

Left ventricular hypertrophy

Left ventricular hypertrophy causes a tall R wave (greater than 25 mm) in V_5 or V_6 and a deep S wave in V_1 or V_2 — but in practice such 'voltage' changes alone are unhelpful in diagnosing left ventricular enlargement. With significant hypertrophy, there are also inverted T waves in I, VL, V_5 and V_6, and sometimes V_4, and there may be left axis deviation. It is difficult to diagnose minor degrees of left ventricular hypertrophy from the ECG.

LEFT VENTRICULAR HYPERTROPHY

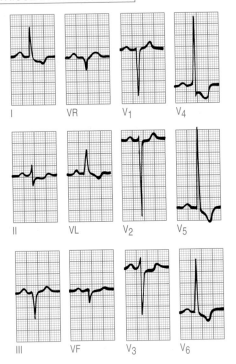

Note: Sinus rhythm

Normal axis (the R and S waves are equal in lead II, so the axis is at the limit of normality)

Height of R wave in V_5 is 35 mm

Deep S waves in V_1 and V_2

Inverted T waves in leads I, VL, V_4–V_6.

The origin of Q waves

Small (septal) 'Q' waves in the left ventricular leads result from depolarization of the septum from left to right (see p. 19). However, Q waves greater than one small square in width (representing 0.04 s), and greater than 2 mm in depth have a quite different significance.

The ventricles are depolarized from inside outwards. Therefore an electrode placed in the cavity of a ventricle would record only a Q wave, because all the depolarization waves would be moving away from it. If a myocardial infarction causes complete death of muscle from the inside surface to the outside surface of the heart, an electrical 'window' is created, and an electrode looking at the heart over that window will record a cavity potential — that is, a Q wave.

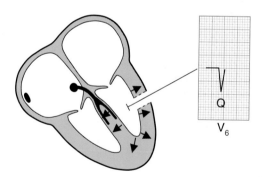

V_6

Q waves greater than one small square in width and at least 2 mm deep therefore indicate a myocardial infarction, and the leads in which the Q wave appears give some indication of the part of the heart that has been damaged.

Thus, infarction of the anterior wall of the left ventricle causes a Q wave in the leads looking at the heart from the front — V_2–V_4 or V_5 (see Ch. 1).

ANTERIOR INFARCTION

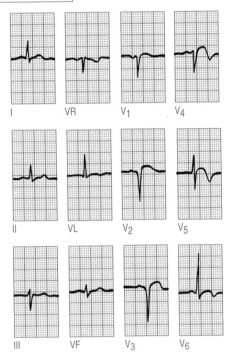

Note: Sinus rhythm
Normal axis
Q waves in leads V_2 and V_3
Inverted T waves in leads V_4–V_6.

If the infarction involves both the anterior and lateral surfaces of the heart, a Q wave will be present in V_3 and V_4 and in the leads that look at the lateral surface — I, VL and V_5–V_6.

ANTERO-LATERAL INFARCTION

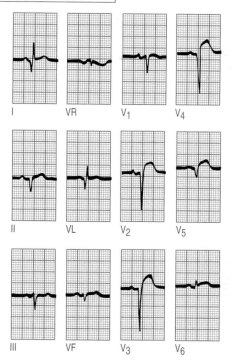

Note: Sinus rhythm

Normal axis (remember that the axis is derived from R and S waves, but not from Q waves)

Q waves in leads I, II, VL, V_3–V_5

Raised ST segments in leads V_2–V_6.

Infarctions of the inferior surface of the heart cause Q waves in the leads looking at the heart from below — III and VF.

INFERIOR INFARCTION

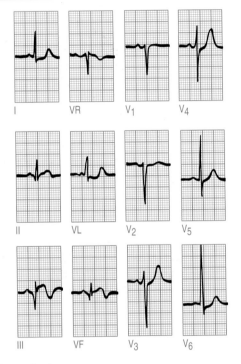

Note: Sinus rhythm
Normal axis
Q waves in leads III and VF
Raised ST segments in leads III and VF
Depressed (ischaemic) ST segments in leads VL and V₆ (see p. 105)
Normal QRS complexes and T waves in the chest leads.

Inferior infarction used to be called 'posterior', but when the posterior wall of the left ventricle is infarcted, a different pattern is seen. The right ventricle occupies the front of the heart anatomically, and normally depolarization of the right ventricle (moving towards the recording electrode V_1) is overshadowed by depolarization of the left ventricle (moving away from V_1). The result is a dominant S wave in V_1 (see Chapter 1). With infarction of the posterior wall of the left ventricle, depolarization of the right ventricle is less opposed by left ventricular forces, and so becomes more obvious and a dominant R wave develops in V_1. The appearance of the ECG is similar to that of right ventricular hypertrophy, though the other changes of right ventricular hypertrophy (see p. 96) do not appear.

The presence of a Q wave does not give any indication of the age of an infarction, because once a Q wave has developed it is usually permanent.

What to do

If the patient gives a story consistent with a myocardial infarction; if the symptoms began less than 12 hours previously; if the ST segments are raised; and if there are no contraindications — treat the patient with a thrombolytic.

ABNORMALITIES OF THE ST SEGMENT

The ST segment lies between the QRS complex and the T wave.

ST segment

It should be 'isoelectric' — that is, at the same level as the part between the T and the next P — but it may be elevated

ST elevated

or depressed.

ST depressed

Elevation of the ST segment is an indication of acute myocardial injury, usually due either to a recent infarction or to pericarditis. The leads in which the elevation occurs indicate the part of the heart that is damaged — anterior damage shows in the V leads, and inferior damage in III and VF. Pericarditis is not usually a localized affair, and so it causes ST elevation in most leads.

Horizontal depression of the ST segment, associated with an upright T wave, is usually a sign of ischaemia as opposed to infarction. When the ECG at rest is normal, ST segment depression may appear during exercise, particularly when effort induces angina.

EXERCISE-INDUCED ISCHAEMIC CHANGES

Rest

Exercise

Note: In the upper (normal) trace, the heart rate is 55 per minute and the ST segments are isoelectric. In the lower trace, the rate is 140 per minute and the ST segments are horizontally depressed.

Downsloping, as opposed to horizontally-depressed, ST segments are usually due to treatment with digoxin (see p. 109).

What to do

Remember that ischaemia can have causes other than coronary disease — for example, anaemia or aortic stenosis. In the absence of such diagnoses, ischaemia is treated with short- and long-acting nitrates, beta-blockers, and calcium-channel blockers.

ABNORMALITIES OF THE T WAVE

The most common abnormality of the T wave is inversion, which is seen in the following circumstances:

1. Normality
2. Ischaemia
3. Ventricular hypertrophy
4. Bundle branch block
5. Digoxin treatment.

Leads adjacent to those showing inverted T waves sometimes show 'biphasic' T waves — initially upright and then inverted.

Normality

The T wave is normally inverted in VR and in V_1 (and in V_2 in young people and also in V_3 in some black people).

Ischaemia

After a myocardial infarction, the first abnormality seen on the ECG is elevation of the ST segment. Subsequently Q waves appear, and the T waves become inverted. The ST segment returns to the baseline, the whole process taking a variable time but usually within the range of 24–48 hours. T wave inversion is often permanent.

DEVELOPMENT OF INFERIOR INFARCTION

1 hour after onset of pain

I   II   III   VR   VL   VF

6 hours after onset of pain

I   II   III   VR   VL   VF

24 hours after onset of pain

I   II   III   VR   VL   VF

Note: Three ECGs have been recorded over 24 hours, and
have been arranged horizontally

Sinus rhythm with a normal cardiac axis in all three
ECGs

The first record is essentially normal

6 hours after the onset of pain, the ST segments
have risen in leads II, III and VF and the ST segment
is depressed in lead VL. A Q wave has developed in
lead III

24 hours after the onset of pain, a small Q wave has

appeared in lead II; the ST segments have returned to baseline, and the T waves are now inverted in leads III and VF.

If an infarction is not full-thickness and so does not cause an electrical window, there will be T wave inversion but no Q waves. This is called a 'non-Q wave infarction' pattern. The term 'subendocardial infarction' pattern is sometimes used, but it is often not pathologically correct.

NON-Q WAVE INFARCTION

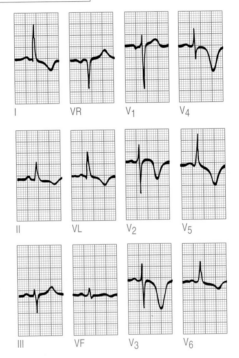

Note: Sinus rhythm
Normal axis
Normal QRS complexes
Inverted T waves in leads I, II, VL, V_2–V_6.

Ventricular hypertrophy

Left ventricular hypertrophy causes inverted T waves in leads looking at the left ventricle (V_5, V_6, II and VL) (see above). Right ventricular hypertrophy causes T wave inversion in the leads looking at the right ventricle (T wave inversion is normal in V_1, but in white adults is abnormal in V_2 or V_3).

Bundle branch block

The abnormal path of depolarization in bundle branch block is usually associated with an abnormal path of repolarization. Therefore, inverted T waves associated with QRS complexes which have a duration of 0.16 s or more have no significance in themselves.

Digoxin

The administration of digoxin causes T wave inversion, characteristically with sloping depression of the ST segment. It is helpful to record an ECG *before* giving digitalis, to save later confusion about the significance of T wave changes.

DIGITALIS EFFECT

Note: Atrial fibrillation
Narrow QRS complexes
Downsloping ST segments ('reversed tick')
Inverted T waves.

OTHER ABNORMALITIES OF THE ST SEGMENT AND THE T WAVE

Electrolyte abnormalities

Abnormalities of the plasma levels of potassium, calcium, and magnesium affect the ECG, though changes in the plasma sodium level do not. The T wave and QT interval (measured from the onset of the QRS complex to the end of the T wave) are most commonly affected.

A low potassium level causes T wave flattening and the appearance of a hump on the end of the T wave called a 'U' wave. A high potassium level causes tall, wide, peaked T waves with the disappearance of the ST segment. The QRS complex may be widened. The effects of abnormal magnesium levels are similar.

A low plasma calcium level causes prolongation of the QT interval, and a high plasma calcium level shortens it.

Non-specific changes

Minor degrees of ST segment and T wave abnormalities (T wave flattening, etc.) are usually of no great significance, and are best reported as 'non-specific ST–T changes'.

ECG INTERPRETATION

Now report on the following four 12-lead ECG records which illustrate various abnormalities.

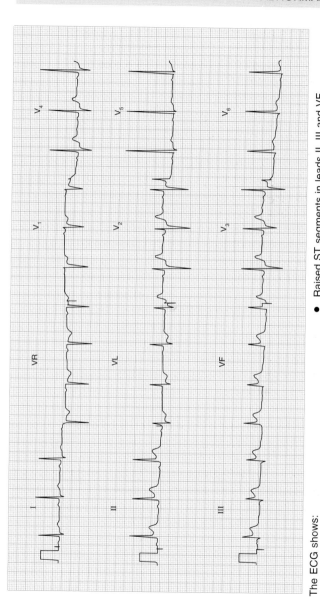

The ECG shows:
- Sinus rhythm
- Normal axis
- Normal QRS complexes
- Raised ST segments in leads II, III and VF
- Inverted T waves in lead VL and in V_1, which is normal.

Interpretation:
Acute inferior infarction; lateral ischaemia.

The ECG shows:
- Sinus rhythm
- Right axis deviation (deep S waves in lead I)
- Dominant R waves in lead V_1
- Deep S waves in lead V_6
- Inverted T waves in leads II, III, VF, V_1–V_4.

Interpretation:
Severe right ventricular hypertrophy.

The ECG shows:

- Sinus rhythm
- Normal axis
- Normal QRS complexes

- Inverted T waves in leads V_3, V_4
- Biphasic T waves in leads V_2 and V_5.

Interpretation:
Anterior non-Q wave infarction.

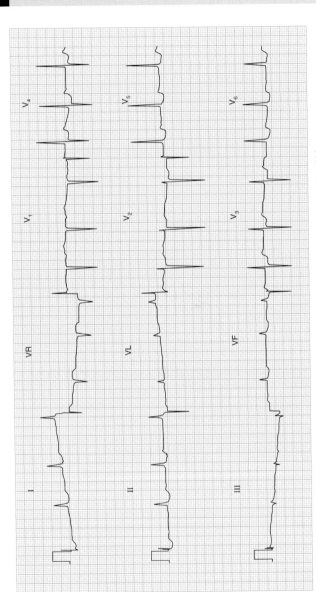

The ECG shows:
- Atrial fibrillation
- Normal axis
- Normal QRS complexes
- Downsloping ST segments, best seen in leads V_4–V_6
- U waves, best seen in lead V_2.

Interpretation:
Atrial fibrillation of uncertain cause, with digitalis effect; U waves suggest hypokalaemia.

THINGS TO REMEMBER

1. Tall P waves result from right atrial hypertrophy, and broad P waves from left atrial hypertrophy.
2. Broadening of the QRS complex indicates abnormal intraventricular conduction: it is seen in bundle branch block and in complexes originating in the ventricular muscle.
3. Increased height of the QRS complex indicates ventricular hypertrophy. Right ventricular hypertrophy is seen in V_1, and left ventricular hypertrophy is seen in V_5 and V_6.
4. Q waves greater than 1 mm across and 2 mm deep indicate myocardial infarction.
5. ST segment elevation indicates acute myocardial infarction or pericarditis.
6. ST segment depression and T wave inversion may be due to ischaemia, ventricular hypertrophy, abnormal intraventricular conduction, or digitalis.
7. T wave inversion is normal in leads III, VR, and V_1. T wave inversion is associated with bundle branch block, ischaemia, and ventricular hypertrophy.
8. T wave flattening or peaking with an unusually long or short QT interval may be due to electrolyte abnormalities, but many minor ST–T changes are non-specific.

And finally, remember

- The ECG is easy to understand.
- Most abnormalities of the ECG are amenable to reason.

CHAPTER 5
Reminders

These lists will remind you of the features that will help you to recognize the patterns of normality and abnormality in the ECG.

WHAT TO LOOK FOR IN THE ECG

1. The rhythm
2. P wave abnormalities:
   peaked, tall — right atrial hypertrophy
   notched, broad — left atrial hypertrophy
3. The cardiac axis
4. The QRS complex:
   width — if wide, ventricular origin or bundle branch block
   height — tall R waves in V_1 in right ventricular hypertrophy
   tall R waves in V_6 in left ventricular hypertrophy
   transition point — R and S waves are equal in the chest lead over the interventricular septum, normally V_3 or V_4; clockwise rotation — chronic lung disease

   Q waves
5. The ST segment:
   raised in acute myocardial infarction and in pericarditis; depressed in ischaemia and with digoxin

6. T waves:
      peaked in hyperkalaemia
      flat, prolonged in hypokalaemia
      inverted:
            normal in some leads
            ischaemia
            infarction
            left or right ventricular hypertrophy
            pulmonary embolism
            bundle branch block
7. U waves:
      can be normal
      hypokalaemia.

THE NORMAL ECG

Limits of normal durations

PR interval: 200 ms (5 small squares)
QRS complex duration: 120 ms (3 small squares)
QT interval: 400 ms (2 large squares).

Rhythm

Sinus arrhythmia
Supraventricular extrasystoles are always normal.

Cardiac axis

Normal axis: QRS complex predominantly upward in I, II, III
              Still normal if QRS complex is downward in III
Right axis: QRS complex predominantly downward in I
Left axis: QRS complex predominantly downward in II
              and III.
NB Minor degrees of right and left axis deviation are within
the normal range.

QRS complex

Small Q waves normal in I, VL, V_6 (septal Qs)
RSR^1 pattern in V_1 normal if duration less than 120 ms
   (partial RBBB)
R wave smaller than S wave in V_1
R wave in V_6 less than 25 mm
R wave in V_6 plus S wave in V_1 less than 35 mm.

ST segment

Should be isoelectric.

T wave

May be inverted in leads:
III
VR
V_1
V_2 and V_3, in Black people.

CONDUCTION PROBLEMS

First degree block

One P wave per QRS complex
PR interval greater than 200 ms.

Second degree block

Wenckebach:	progressive PR lengthening then non-conducted P wave, and then repetition of the cycle
Mobitz Type 2:	occasional non-conducted beats
2:1 (or 3:1) block:	two (or three) P waves per QRS complex, normal P wave rate.

Third degree (complete) block

No relationship between P waves and QRS complexes
Usually, wide QRS complexes
Usual QRS complex rate less than 50 per minute
Sometimes narrow QRS complexes, rate 50–60 per minute.

Right bundle branch block

QRS complex duration greater than 120 ms
RSR^1 pattern
Usually, dominant R^1 wave in V_1
Inverted T waves in V_1, and sometimes in V_2–V_3
Deep and wide S waves in V_6.

Left bundle branch block

QRS complex duration greater than 120 ms
M pattern in V_6, and sometimes in V_4–V_5
No septal Q waves
Inverted T waves in I, VL, V_5–V_6, and sometimes V_4.

Bifascicular block

Left anterior hemiblock (i.e. marked left axis with deep S
    waves in II and III)
Right bundle branch block (see above).

RHYTHMS

Supraventricular rhythms

In general have:
    Narrow QRS complexes (less than 120 ms)
    Same QRS complexes as in sinus rhythm
    Normal T waves.

Exceptions: supraventricular rhythms have wide QRS complexes with:
> bundle branch block
> Wolff-Parkinson-White syndrome.

Ventricular rhythms

In general have:
> Wide QRS complexes (greater than 120 ms)
> Different QRS complexes from those seen in sinus rhythm
> Abnormal T waves.

Rhythm abnormalities

Extrasystoles: single early beats suppressing the next sinus beat
Escape beats: absence of sinus beat followed by late single beat
Tachycardias
Bradycardias.

Common supraventricular rhythms

Sinus rhythm
Atrial extrasystoles
Junctional (AV nodal) extrasystoles
Atrial tachycardia
Atrial flutter
Atrial fibrillation
Junctional (AV nodal) tachycardia
Junctional (AV nodal) escape.

Common ventricular rhythms

Ventricular extrasystoles
Ventricular tachycardia
Ventricular escape (single beats or complete heart block)
Ventricular fibrillation.

Supraventricular rhythms

1. *Sinus rhythm:*
   One P wave per QRS complex
   P–P interval varies with respiration (sinus arrhythmia).
2. *Supraventricular extrasystoles:*
   Early QRS complex
   No P wave, or abnormally-shaped (atrial) P wave
   Narrow and normal QRS complex
   Normal T wave
   Next P wave is 'reset'.
3. *Atrial tachycardia:*
   QRS complex rate greater than 150 per min
   Abnormal P waves, usually with short PR intervals
   Usually one P wave per QRS complex, but sometimes P
     wave rate 200–240 per minute, with 2:1 block.
4. *Atrial flutter:*
   P wave rate 300 per minute
   Sawtoothed pattern
   2:1, 3:1 or 4:1 block
   Block increased by carotid sinus pressure.
5. *Atrial fibrillation:*
   The most irregular rhythm of all
   QRS complex rate characteristically over 160 per minute
     without treatment, but can be slower
   No P waves identifiable, but there is a varying,
     completely irregular baseline.
6. *Junctional (AV nodal) tachycardia:*
   Commonly, but inappropriately, called 'SVT'
     (supraventricular tachycardia)
   No P waves
   Rate usually 150–180 per minute
   Carotid sinus pressure may cause reversion to sinus
     rhythm.
7. *Escape rhythms:*
   Bradycardias, but otherwise characteristics as above,

except that atrial fibrillation does not occur as an escape rhythm.

Ventricular rhythms

1. *Ventricular extrasystoles:*
   Early QRS complex
   No P wave
   QRS complex wide (greater than 120 ms)
   Abnormally-shaped QRS complex
   Abnormally-shaped T wave
   Next P wave is on time.
2. *Ventricular tachycardia:*
   No P waves
   QRS complex rate greater than 160 per minute
   Accelerated idioventricular rhythm: as for ventricular tachycardia, but QRS complex rate less than 120 per minute.
3. *Ventricular fibrillation:*
   Look at the patient, not the ECG.

MYOCARDIAL INFARCTION

Sequence of ECG changes

1. Normal ECG
2. Raised ST segments
3. Appearance of Q waves
4. Normalization of ST segments
5. Inversion of T waves.

Site of infarction

Anterior infarction: changes classically in V_3–V_4, but
                         often also in V_2–V_5
Inferior infarction: changes in III and VF

Lateral infarction: changes in I, VL, V_5–V_6
True posterior infarction: dominant R waves in V_1.

PULMONARY EMBOLISM

Possible ECG patterns include:
Normal ECG with sinus tachycardia
Peaked P waves
Right axis deviation
Right bundle branch block
Dominant R waves in V_1 (i.e. R wave bigger than S wave)
Inverted T waves in leads V_1–V_3
Deep S waves in lead V_6
Right axis (S waves in I), plus Q waves and inverted T
    waves in III.

HYPERTROPHY OF THE HEART

Right ventricular hypertrophy

Tall R waves in V_1
T wave inversion in V_1 and V_2, and sometimes in V_3 and
    even V_4
Deep S waves in V_6
Right axis deviation
Sometimes, RBBB.

Left ventricular hypertrophy

R waves in V_5 or V_6 greater than 25 mm
R waves in V_5 or V_6 plus S waves in V_1 or V_2 greater than
    35 mm
Inverted T waves in I, VL, V_5–V_6, and sometimes V_4.

Left atrial hypertrophy

Bifid P waves.

Right atrial hypertrophy

Peaked P waves.

DIFFERENTIAL DIAGNOSIS OF ECG CHANGES

We can rearrange some of these lists to remind you of the possible implications of ECG patterns.

P:QRS apparently not 1:1

If you cannot see one P wave per QRS complex, consider the following:

1. P wave present but not easily visible: look particularly at II and V_1
2. If QRS complexes are irregular, rhythm is probably atrial fibrillation and what seem to be P waves actually are not
3. If QRS complex rate is rapid and there are no P waves, a wide QRS complex indicates ventricular tachycardia and a narrow QRS complex indicates junctional (AV nodal) tachycardia
4. If QRS complex rate is slow, it is probably an escape rhythm.

P:QRS more than 1:1

If you can see more P waves than QRS complexes, consider the following:

1. If the P wave rate is 300 per minute, the rhythm is atrial flutter
2. If the P wave rate is 150–200 per minute and there are two Q waves per QRS complex, the rhythm is atrial tachycardia with block
3. If the P wave rate is normal (say, 60–100 per minute) and there is 2:1 conduction, the rhythm is sinus with second degree block

4. If the PR interval appears to be different with each beat, complete (third degree) heart block is probably present.

Wide QRS complexes (greater than 120 ms)

Wide QRS complexes are characteristic of:
Sinus rhythm with bundle branch block
Sinus rhythm with Wolff-Parkinson-White syndrome
Ventricular extrasystoles
Ventricular tachycardia
Complete heart block.

Q waves

Small (septal) normal in I, VL, V_6
Q waves in III but not VF is a normal variant
Probably indicate infarction if present in more than one
   lead, longer than 40 ms in duration, and deeper than 2 mm
Q waves in III but not in VF, with right axis, may indicate
   pulmonary embolus
Leads showing Q waves indicate site of infarction.

ST segment depression

Digoxin: ST segment slopes downwards
Ischaemia: flat ST depression.

T wave inversion

Normal in III, VR, V_1, V_2–V_3 in Black people
Ventricular rhythms
Bundle branch block
Myocardial infarction
Right or left ventricular hypertrophy
Wolff-Parkinson-White syndrome.

Index

Accelerated idioventricular rhythm, 63
Acute infarction, 104
Anterior infarction, 100
Antero-lateral infarction, 101
Arrhythmia
    reminders, 119–122
    sinus, 54
    treatment, 90–91
Atrial escape rhythm, 59
Atrial extrasystole, 65
Atrial fibrillation, 78–79, 121
Atrial flutter, 71–73, 121
    with 2:1 block, 72
    with carotid sinus pressure, 73
Atrial hypertrophy
    left, 93
    right, 93, 96
Atrial tachycardia, 70
Atrioventricular block, 28, 71
Atrioventricular (AV) node, 2, 6, 27
    conduction problems, 28–32
Axis
    cardiac, 14, 43, 116
    deviation
        right, 15, 96
        left, 16, 44
    normal, 14, 44

Bifascicular block, 45, 119
Bilateral bundle branch block, 33
Block
    atrioventricular, 28, 71
    bifascicular, 46

bundle branch, 33–42, 76
    bilateral, 33
    left, 34, 38, 40, 42, 119
    right, 34, 35, 37, 41, 45, 119
    and T wave, 109
fascicular, left anterior, 44
heart block, 28–32
    first degree, 28–29, 118
    second degree, 29–32, 118
        2:1, 31, 32
        3:1, 31
    third degree (complete), 32, 63,
        119
hemiblock, left anterior, 44
Bundle, accessory, 81
Bundle branch block, 33–52
    bilateral, 33
    left, 34, 38–40, 42
    right, 34, 35–37, 41, 45
        and left axis deviation, 45
    and T wave, 109
Bundle of His, 2, 5
    conduction problems and AV
        node, 28–32

Calibration, ECG recorder, 11
Cardiac axis, 14, 43, 117
Carotid sinus pressure, 73
Complete (third degree) heart
    block, 32, 63
Conduction problems, 27–52, 118–119
    in AV node and His bundle, 28–32
    bundle branches, 33–52

Definitions, QRS complex, 4
Delta wave, 81
Depolarization, 2, 12, 13, 27, 33
Digoxin (digitalis), and T wave, 109
Differential diagnosis of ECG
        changes, 124

ECG recorder, 5–11, 116–118
    12-lead, 8
    calibration, 11
    times and speeds, 5–6
Ectopic beat, 64
Electrolyte abnormalities and T wave, 110
Enhanced automaticity, 83
Escape rhythm, 57–62, 121–122
    atrial, 59
    junctional, 60
    ventricular, 61–62
Exercise and ischaemia, 105
Extrasystoles, 64–69
    atrial, 65
    junctional, 65
    supraventricular, 68, 121
    ventricular, 66–69, 122

Fascicles of left bundle branch, 43
Fibrillation
    atrial, 78–79
    ventricular, 80
First degree heart block, 28–29, 118

Heart block, 28–32
    first degree, 28–29, 118
    second degree, 29–32, 118
        with atrial flutter, 72
        causes of, 32
        Mobitz Type 2, 29, 32
        Wenckebach, 30, 32
        2:1, 31, 32
        3:1, 31
    third degree (complete), 32, 63, 119
Hemiblock, left anterior, 44
Hypertrophy, 93–98, 123–124
    atrial
        left, 93, 123
        right, 93, 96, 124
    ventricular
        left, 97–98, 123

    right, 95–97, 123
    and T wave, 109

Infarction, site, 122–123
Inferior infarction, 102
    development of, 107
Ischaemia, 105–106
    and exercise, 105
    and T wave, 106

Junctional escape rhythm, 60
Junctional extrasystole, 65
Junctional tachycardia, 74

Lead, 7
Left anterior fascicular block, 44
Left anterior hemiblock, 44
Left axis deviation, 16, 38
Left bundle branch block, 34, 38–40,
        42

Mitral stenosis, 93
Mobitz Type 2 phenomenon, 29, 32
Myocardial infarction, 99–108, 122–123
    acute, 104
    anterior, 100
    antero-lateral, 101
    inferior, 102
        development of, 107
    subendocardial, 108

Nodal see Junctional
Normal axis, 14, 44

P wave
    abnormalities, 93
    bifid, 93
    broad, 93
    tall, 7
Pericardial effusion, 11
PR interval, 6, 28
    prolonged, 28
    short, 81
Pre-excitation, 81
Premature contraction, 64
Pulmonary embolism, 97, 123
Pulmonary hypertension, 95, 96
Purkinje fibres, 3

Q wave, septal, 19, 94
Q waves, 9
  origin, 99
QRS
  duration, 6
  shape, 12
    in V leads, 18
QRS complex
  abnormalities, 94–103
  definition, 4, 118
  widening, 33

R on T phenomenon, 66
R wave, tall, 11
Re-entry, 81
  tachycardia, 83
Reminders, 116–125
Repolarization, 3
Right axis deviation, 15, 96
Right bundle branch block, 34
  35–37, 41, 45
  and left axis deviation, 45
Rhythm, 53–91
  abnormal, treatment of, 90–91
  accelerated idioventricular, 63
  escape, 57–62
    atrial, 59
    junctional, 60
    ventricular, 61–62
  intrinsic, 53–54
  sinus, 53, 74
    with left bundle branch
      block, 76
  supraventricular, 55–56
  ventricular, 56

S wave, 20
Second degree heart block, 29–31
  2:1, 31, 32
  with atrial flutter, 72
  causes of, 32
  Mobitz Type 2, 29, 32
  Wenckebach, 30, 32
Sinoatrial (SA) node, 2, 27
Sinus arrhythmia, 54
Sinus bradycardia, 54

Sinus rhythm, 54, 74
  with left bundle branch
    block, 76
Sinus tachycardia, 55
Subendocardial infarction, 108
Supraventricular extrasystole, 68
Supraventricular rhythm, 55–56
Supraventricular tachycardia, 70

T wave
  abnormalities, 106–110
  and bundle branch block, 109
  changes, non-specific, 110
  and digoxin, 109
  and electrolyte abnormalities, 110
  and ischaemia, 106
  and ventricular hypertrophy, 109
Tachycardia, 70–77
  atrial, 70, 121
  junctional, 74
  re-entry, 83
  sinus, 55
  supraventricular, 70
  treatment, first line, 91
  ventricular, 75, 122
Third degree (complete) heart block,
  32, 63
Times and speeds, ECG recorder, 5–7
Transition point, 22

Vagus nerves, 54
Ventricular escape rhythm, 61–62
Ventricular extrasystole, 66–69
Ventricular fibrillation, 80, 122
Ventricular hypertrophy
  left, 98
  right, 95–97
  and T wave, 109
Ventricular rhythm, 56, 122
Ventricular tachycardia, 75, 122

Wenckebach phenomenon, 30, 32
Window, electrical, 99
Wolff-Parkinson-White (WPW)
        syndrome, 81–83

Your COMPLETE Guide to the ECG

The ECG Made Easy

John R Hampton

July 1997   0 443 05681 1
International Edition available: 0443 05695 1

This popular text provides a readable guide to ECG interpretation, with an emphasis throughout on straightforward practical application. Whatever your clinical role, make sure you have the ideal pocket reference to this essential diagnostic tool!

"ideal for students wishing to learn the basic essentials of electrocardiography ... good value for money."

Mediscope

"a godsend to thousands of practising physicians and surgeons who never really mastered the ECG but always felt that they should have done."

European Medical Journal

The ECG in Practice
3rd edition
John R Hampton

July 1997   0 443 05680 3

Although the ECG is easy in principle, variations in its pattern can make it seem complex. **The ECG in Practice** is a companion volume to **The ECG Made Easy**. It has been written to help you make the most of the ECG – and to appreciate its limitations.

"the pocket reference for junior doctors."

Nursing Standard

"an excellent book for medical students and junior medical staff."

Cardiovascular Research

100 ECG Problems

John R Hampton

July 1997   0 443 05678 1

There is no substitute for reporting a large number of ECGs. This book provides 100 real clinical case histories, with the 12-lead ECG from each patient. You are asked to report and interpret each ECG, and to draw up a plan for the patient's management. The answers are given on the reverse of the page showing the ECG.